Visual Development

PERSPECTIVES IN VISION RESEARCH

Series Editor: Colin Blakemore
University of Oxford
Oxford, England

A Continuation Order Plan is available for this series. A continuation order will bring delivery of each new volume immediately upon publication. Volumes are billed only upon actual shipment. For further information please contact the publisher.

Visual Development

Nigel W. Daw

Yale University Medical School
New Haven, Connecticut

Plenum Press · New York and London

Library of Congress Cataloging-in-Publication Data

Daw, Nigel.
    Visual development / Nigel W. Daw.
        p.   cm. -- (Perspectives in vision research)
    Includes bibliographical references and index.
    ISBN 0-306-45023-2
    1. Vision. 2. Developmental biology. 3. Eyes--Growth.
4. Amblyopia.   I. Title. II. Series.
    [DNLM: 1. Visual Pathways--growth & development. 2. Vision
Disorders-- physiopathology. 3. Vision--physiology. 4. Neuronal
Plasticity--physiology.   WW 103 D269v 1995]
    QP475.D35 1995
    612.8'4--dc20
DNLM/DLC
for Library of Congress   95-32577
                                                                    CIP

ISBN 0-306-45023-2

© 1995 Plenum Press, New York
A Division of Plenum Publishing Corporation
233 Spring Street, New York, N. Y. 10013

10 9 8 7 6 5 4 3 2

Printed in the United States of America

Foreword

The transformation in our understanding of the development of vision over the past 30 years or so has been quite remarkable. Three lines of evidence once poles apart—clinical, behavioral, and neurobiological—have now converged and reinforced each other. Nigel Daw's book documents that meeting of methodologies, which has so radically advanced our knowledge of how vision develops and how that development can go wrong.

The fundamental issue was and remains, of course, the ancient one of Nature versus Nurture: Are our extraordinary visual capacities purely dependent on innate mechanisms, or are they partly sculpted by experience?

In the early 1960s, the clearest evidence for an influence of visual experience on visual development came from the clinic. For 200 years ophthalmologists had known that disturbances of visual experience could lead to inferior visual ability later on. The condition of developmental *amblyopia* was and remains the most potent testimony that what we are able to see in adult life is influenced by what and how we saw when we were young. Amblyopia—literally blunted vision—is defined as abnormally low visual acuity, usually in one eye, even with optimal refractive correction and in the absence of any obvious retinal or central pathology. But the deficit in vision in amblyopia is far more than a reduction in the ability to resolve fine detail. Most amblyopes have reduced sensitivity to contrast over part of the range of spatial size, and they often describe the image through the affected eye as confused or scrambled. Amblyopia is a very common condition affecting perhaps as many as 3% of the population (depending on its quantitative definition). Monocular developmental amblyopia is apparently inevitably associated with one of three predisposing conditions: deprivation of vision (through ptosis of the eyelid, cataract, corneal opacity, etc.); habitual defocus in one eye (through anisometropia, i.e., a difference in refractive state in the two eyes); or convergent strabismus or squint (although amblyopia is very rare in divergent squint).

With hindsight, routine clinical observations can now be interpreted in terms of concepts that have been established through experimental work on animals and human amblyopes. First, although binocular deprivation or defocus can result in bilateral amblyopia, it is clear that the risk is much greater if the quality of vision is compromised in only one eye; in current parlance, *competitive* forces must be at work. Although it was realized that this kind of amblyopia never occurs *de novo* in adult life, the notion of a *sensitive period* for the influences of disordered visual experience arose through studies of carefully controlled manipulation or deprivation of vision in animals. Indeed, the rigorous experimental approach to amblyopia, which is the thread that runs through the whole of this book, has not only produced results and ideas of fundamental importance to developmental neuroscience but has also illuminated and clarified clinical dilemmas.

A glance at any textbook of ophthalmology of the 1950s will demonstrate how substantially our understanding of amblyopia has advanced since that time. At that stage even the predisposing conditions were not known for certain. The variety of "treatments," some bizarre, none of them very effective, was a strong indication of ignorance. And theories of the nature and site of the fundamental pathology underlying amblyopia were pure speculation: As many experts thought that it was likely to be retinal in origin as believed it to be a central disorder.

In the mid 1960s, largely as a result of the pioneering work of T. N. Wiesel and D. H. Hubel, basic understanding of the functional organization of the visual system marched ahead, and with it came the opportunity for a rational attack on the problem of amblyopia and an experimental approach to the Nature–Nurture question. A seminal contribution was a paper published in 1963 that showed that neurons of the primary visual cortex of the cat, which are normally capable of being activated by stimulation of either eye, lose their functional input from one eye if that eye has been deprived by closing the lids early in life (Wiesel, T. N., & Hubel, D. H., 1963, Single cell responses in striate cortex of kittens deprived of vision in one eye. *J. Neurophysiol.* **26:** 1003–1017). Since an equal period of binocular deprivation leaves most cells still responsive, the interpretation was that afferent axons carrying signals into the cortex from the two eyes are competing for influence on cortical neurons. Subsequent work has revealed the exact conditions required for normal postnatal maturation of the visual cortex, the many aspects of neuronal selectivity that can be affected by different forms of deprivation, and the nature, duration, and varieties of sensitive periods during which activity and deprivation influence normal development. Synaptic plasticity, activity-dependence, self-organization, coincidence detection, and neural network learning—all these concepts, so central to current thinking about the cerebral cortex, have grown largely out of studies of development and modification of the visual system.

As neurobiological approaches provided more and more information about normal development of the visual pathway and about activity-dependent processes, techniques became available for asking exact and rigorous questions about the visual capabilities of young animals, including humans. The introduction of the preferential looking method gave behavioral psychologists a tool with which to probe early powers of detection and discrimination and the way in which they mature.

Nigel Daw, who has himself made important contributions to studies of selective deprivation and the nature of sensitive periods, reviews this complicated and controversial field in this volume and attempts to relate experimental findings to clinical issues. Rational accounts of the locus and basis of amblyopia can now be given, leading to clear views about the importance of early diagnosis and corrective procedures.

As knowledge of normal development and the way in which it can be subverted by deprivation of experience have advanced, many of the questions have focused on the fundamental cellular and molecular mechanisms that underlie synaptic plasticity and activity dependence in the visual cortex. Daw provides an incisive and critical review of this topical field and concentrates on the evidence for involvement of the NMDA glutamate receptor in mediating synaptic learning and visual plasticity, another area where he himself has made important contributions.

This important book, unique in the breadth of its coverage, will be of interest to a wide range of researchers and students in both the basic and the clinical sciences.

Colin Blakemore

University of Oxford
Oxford, England

Preface

Research in the area of visual development has become a multidisciplinary affair. Students who acquire an interest in the field therefore need to understand several different aspects of the subject. The development of acuity measured by psychophysicists is the concern of optometrists and ophthalmologists, and it depends on changes in the anatomy of the retina and the physiology of cells in the visual pathway. Scientists working on the cellular, molecular, and biochemical mechanisms rely on anatomical studies, physiology, and psychophysics in designing and interpreting their experiments. Indeed, the laboratories of all of the leading scientists working in the field now employ a large variety of techniques in their studies.

Because the study of visual development is pursued by workers in many disciplines, from medicine to basic science, I have tried to write this book at a level that can be understood by students from different disciplines: graduate students in neurobiology and psychology as well as optometry students and ophthalmology residents. The text assumes some knowledge of basic terms, but a glossary is provided should the reader encounter some words that are unfamiliar. The emphasis is on facts and conclusions, rather than on methods and procedures.

I hope that experts will also read the book. The subject has become so wide-ranging that not many people have the time to read the literature in all of its aspects. The book is also intended for experts in one area to get a grasp of the basics of the subject in other disciplines that are not their primary discipline.

To write a book covering so many disciplines, I have had to simplify. The book does not go into controversies in detail. Instead, it provides my summary of what seems to me to be the best evidence. Not everyone will agree with my synthesis. Some experts will read it and be outraged at some of my statements. However, my outrageous statements were intended to be constructive: I hope that they will provoke thought and point the way to more experiments that will carry the field forward.

I am grateful to Colin Blakemore for inviting me to write this book and for commenting on it. The process has been an educational one for me, and it has led to a number of insights that may have been apparent to others, but not to me. A number of friends and colleagues have helped me in the book's preparation.

In particular, Grace Gray read the entire text twice and improved it throughout. Robert Hess went through the whole section on Visual Deprivation and made many valuable comments. John Lisman did the same for the section on Mechanisms. Janette Atkinson, Marty Banks, Oliver Braddick, Jan Naegele, Pasko Rakic, and Josh Wallman read individual chapters in their area of expertise and made many corrections and improvements. Several of my colleagues in the Department of Ophthalmology—Ethan Cohen, Jonathan Kirsch, Marvin Sears, Thomas Hughes, Colin Barnstable, Silvia Reid, and Helen Flavin—gave comments on various portions of the text, and Marc Weitzman read two whole sections. I would like to thank them all. However, I did not adopt all of their suggestions, and the errors and omissions are mine. I would also like to thank John Woolsey for the preparation of several figures and Janet Hescock and Bob Brown for help in the preparation of the text and photographs, together with support from the Core Grant to the Department of Ophthalmology and Visual Science at Yale University from the National Eye Institute.

Contents

Chapter 4

Anatomical Development of the Visual System

Chapter 5

Development of Receptive Field Properties

Section II

Amblyopia and the Effects of Visual Deprivation

Chapter 6

**Modifications to the Visual Input That Lead to Nervous
System Changes**

Chapter 7

Physiological and Anatomical Changes That Result from Optical and Motor Deficits

Chapter 8

What Is Amblyopia?

Chapter 9

Critical Periods

Section III

Mechanisms of Plasticity

Chapter 10

Concepts of Plasticity

Chapter 11

Long-Term Potentiation as a Model

Chapter 12

Mechanisms of Plasticity in the Visual Cortex

Chapter 13

Deprivation Myopia and Emmetropization

Section IV

Conclusions

Chapter 14

Future Studies

1

Introduction

Visual deprivation is an important and fascinating subject from several points of view: clinical, philosophical, historical, and scientific. Many general questions in these areas have been framed over the years in terms of the visual system. This is not surprising, because we are visual animals. If dogs ruled the world, the title of this book would be *Olfactory Development*. As it is, vision is the most important sense to us, and the first that we think of in discussing scientific and philosophical questions.

There are a large number of people who have personally experienced some form of visual deprivation. Anything that affects the images on the retinas of young children can have lasting effects on the part of the brain that processes visual signals. This can occur if one eye is in focus, but the other is not; if vertical lines are in focus, but horizontal lines are not; if the two eyes look in different directions (strabismus); if the lens of one or both eyes is cloudy (cataract); or if the eyeball grows so much that objects can no longer be focused on the retina. Frequently these conditions lead to poor vision in one or both eyes as a result of changes that have occurred in the central visual system, even after the images on the retinas are made clear and coordinated. The Greeks named this poor vision *amblyopia*, meaning blunt vision, or dull vision. The colloquial term for amblyopia is *lazy eye*. Between 2 and 4% of the population may become amblyopic from visual deprivation.

Philosophers became interested in the subject of visual deprivation when William Molyneux posed his famous question in the late 17th century. After his wife became blind, Molyneux wrote to John Locke: "Suppose a man born blind, and now adult, and taught by his touch to distinguish between a cube and a sphere of the same metal. . . . Suppose then the cube and sphere placed on a table and the blind man made to see; query, Whether by his sight, before he touched them, he could now distinguish and tell which is the globe, and which the cube? To which the acute and judicious proposer answers: not. For though he has obtained the experience of how a globe, how a cube, affects his touch, yet he has not yet attained the experience that what affects his touch so or so, must affect his sight so or so."

Locke's reply in 1690 was that "I agree with this thinking gentleman, whom I am proud to call my friend, in his answer to this his problem, and am of opinion that the blind man, at first sight, would not be able with certainty to say which was the globe, which the cube whilst he only saw them; though he could unerringly name them by his touch, and certainly distinguish them by the difference of their figures felt" (see Locke, 1846).

Some material to test Molyneux's question was available during his time. Congenital cataract was quite common, and an operation for it called couching had been invented in either Arabia or India at least 1000 years earlier (Hirschberg, 1982). A sharp needle was used to make a hole in the sclera, then a blunt needle was inserted, and the lens gently pushed downward out of the line of sight. Occasionally the cataract was removed altogether with a hollow needle, but not many surgeons were expert enough to do this well. Thus, the operation was often not successful. Moreover, vision was not fully restored because of lack of adequate correction for the absent lens. Consequently, the topic of Molyneux's question remained an armchair discussion for another half century.

Substantial numbers of patients with clear restored vision resulted only when physicians finally realized that the cataract is in the lens, and Daviel promulgated a cleaner operation for cataract by removing the lens through a flap in the cornea. Generally speaking, the results of this operation were successful in producing a clear image on the retina, when spectacles were worn, but were disappointing to the patients in terms of their visual perception. Daviel stated in 1762 after 22 cases, "I can assert, indeed, with absolute assurance, that not a single one of these patients has recognized the objects shown to him after the operation, without the use of touch, unless they have been many times shown to him and named. . . . If it has been said that some such patients can distinguish objects exactly and completely immediately after the operation, then this shows that they were not really blind from birth, for the latter have no real idea at all of even the meanest objects" (von Senden, 1960, p. 106).

Numerous cases were reported following Daviel, and the results were generally the same. von Senden collected them in a summary in 1932 (von Senden, tr. 1960). Where vision was tested soon after the operation, patients could distinguish color, but they had little idea of form or shape, no idea of distance, no idea of depth, and very little idea of solidity. Their problem was not just a matter of transferring the recognition of objects by touch to the recognition of objects by sight. Their visual perception in itself was defective. Frequently they became depressed because the gift of sight was confusing for them (von Senden, 1960; Gregory, 1974). They could not, in fact, see like normal people, and their previous tactual and auditory world was not easily correlated with their new visual world.

Locke was the apostle of empiricism. He believed that everything is learned. The opposing point of view is that everything is innate. The debate between the two points of view raged for many years under various headings, such as nature, for the belief that properties are with us at birth, versus nurture, for the belief that properties are learned from experience after birth. One might think, from the cases discussed by von Senden, that Locke's point of view is correct. As we will discuss, neither point of view is strictly correct. While some properties are learned, others are present at birth. Moreover (an answer to Molyneux's question that Locke did not consider), properties can be present at birth and then degenerate.

The history of strabismus (i.e., being cross-eyed or squinting) is as venerable as that of cataract. Hippocrates (460–375 B.C.) believed there was a genetic component, saying that "if, therefore, bald persons have for the most part bald children, grey-eyed parents grey-eyed children, squinting parents squinting children, and so on . . ." (see Hippocrates, tr. 1923). Paulus of Aegina (625–690) recommended wearing a mask with "an opening for each eye so placed as to induce the eyes to assume direct positions in order to see through these openings." Georg Bartisch (1535–1606) illustrates such a mask for convergent strabismus, together with a mask containing prisms for divergent strabismus (Fig. 1.1).

Surgery for strabismus was initially attempted by Chevalier John Taylor in the 18th century (Albert, 1992). It is not clear exactly what the surgery entailed. Many of his operations were not successful: he treated Johann Sebastian Bach twice, and Bach went blind afterward. However, Taylor was a colorful personality who gave great publicity to the possibility of surgery for the problem. The first successful surgery is attributed to Johann Freidrich Dieffenbach (1792–1847), although others attempted it, some successfully, around the same date. In the early days, the operation was performed as much for cosmetic as for visual effect. From ancient times strabismus was associated with an "evil eye," and people who had it were frequently treated with suspicion, like the village idiot. They were more concerned about the ridicule and shame from their crooked eye than any visual problems caused by it.

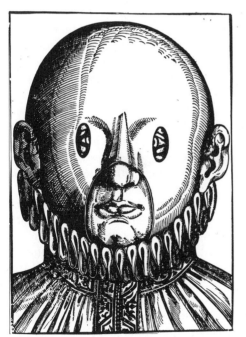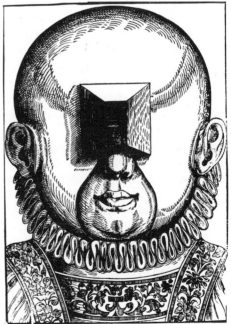

FIG. 1.1. Masks for squinters. On the left is a mask for a convergent squinter with holes placed to try to force the eyes to look outward. On the right is a mask for divergent squinters containing two prisms that will make the images converge. From Bartisch (1583).

Indeed, surgery for strabismus, like surgery for cataract, can be a disappointment to the patient. In a few cases, the crooked eye establishes a compensating point of fixation away from the fovea that is coordinated with the normal point of fixation at the fovea in the good eye, and the operation can lead to double vision. The double vision can be much more disturbing than the amblyopia in the "lazy eye" that was there before the operation.

If treatment is to be successful for cataract or strabismus acquired early in life, and disappointment is to be avoided, the treatment must be started early. This point was not fully appreciated until the middle of the 20th century. A nonsurgical treatment for amblyopia in strabismus (patching of the good eye) was recommended by Buffon in 1743. However, this treatment fell into disrepute, and almost 200 years passed before it became apparent that it could be successful in young children, but not older children (von Noorden, 1990). Slowly ophthalmologists turned from the idea that strabismus is a congenital defect to the idea that it is also a developmental defect (von Noorden, 1990; Tychsen, 1993). This latter idea led to the recognition of the importance of early intervention, and to the concept of a critical period after which intervention would be unsuccessful.

The modern period in the investigation of visual deprivation started with the work of Torsten Wiesel and David Hubel in the early 1960s, for which they were awarded the Nobel prize in 1981 (Wiesel, 1982). It was this work that enabled the behavioral observations made in the clinic to be correlated with physiological and anatomical changes that occur in the central visual system. Several technical advances contributed to this work. First, there was the invention of the microelectrode, which allowed investigation of the properties of single cells in the visual system. Second, there was the development of an anatomical method for demonstrating the endings of axons projecting from the eyes to the visual cortex. Third, there was the development of techniques for visualizing how cells in the cortex that have similar properties are grouped together.

These experiments demonstrated that the main site for changes occurring after visual deprivation is the primary visual cortex. Projections to the primary visual cortex change. Properties of cells in the visual cortex change. Connections between cells in the visual cortex change. In other words, sensory signals carried from the eye to the brain have a dramatic effect on the structure and physiological properties of the brain.

More recently, the focus has moved to the biochemical steps occurring in these events. Many suggestions as to what these steps might be come from work on "long-term potentiation." This is a phenomenon that has been studied in the hippocampus as well as the visual cortex, and is believed to underlie memory, primarily because it occurs in the hippocampus at all ages, and lesions of the hippocampus are known to disrupt memory.

This book will trace the main themes in this story. The first section will summarize the psychophysical properties, the anatomy, and the physiology of normal development of the visual system. An important component of this section will be to point out which aspects of development depend on sensory signals, and which do not. There is considerable development after birth. Indeed, acuity in an infant is sufficiently poor (less than 10% of normal adult acuity) that a newborn infant is legally blind by adult criteria. Thus, the effects of visual deprivation will depend on when in development the deprivation occurs.

The second section will deal with the behavioral, physiological, and anatomical effects of visual deprivation. This section will present a summary of the clinical literature on the subject, and also the basic science literature from experiments on animals. Then, the clinical and basic research findings will be correlated with each other to provide insights into the basic mechanisms of the human pathology resulting from visual deprivation.

The third section will deal with mechanisms of visual deprivation. Here we are addressing our understanding of deprivation as it unfolds. The sensory signals that reach the visual cortex have long-term effects that eventually lead to anatomical changes. There must be a number of intermediate steps between the sensory signals and the anatomical changes. The steps are beginning to be understood. Moreover, some of the steps are present in young animals and relatively absent in adults, and it is these steps that make the visual cortex of young animals more able to adapt to the signals coming in. However, there is a lot more to be discovered. This is a very active area of research at the moment. This section of the book will probably be the first to go out of date.

The story has come a long way since Molyneux set down his question. There have been both philosophical and practical developments. The realization that there are innate properties in the visual cortex that can degenerate in the absence of proper visual input has led ophthalmologists to intervene earlier and earlier. The knowledge of ophthalmologists that treatment of cataract is much less likely to be successful than treatment of strabismus, and that treatment of strabismus may bring back acuity but not stereopsis, has led basic scientists to measure the critical periods for development of these features more accurately. There have been few books that bring together the various aspects of the story, and none at the level of this book, so I hope that the publication of this book will foster yet more interactions in the field.

References

Albert, D. M., 1992, Introduction, in: *The Muscles of the Eye* (L. Howe, ed.), Gryphon Editions, Delran, NJ, pp. 3–30.

Bartisch, G., 1583, *Ophthalmodouleia, das ist augendienst*, Stockel, Dresden.

Buffon, M. de, 1743, Dissertation sur la cause du strabisme ou les yeux louches, *Hist. Acad. R. Sci.* 231–248.

Gregory, R. L., 1974, *Concepts and Mechanisms of Perception*, Scribner's, New York, pp. 65–129.

Hippocrates, 1923, Air, Water and Places, in: *Collected Works* (W. H. S. Jones, ed.), William Heinemann, London, p. 111.

Hirschberg, J., 1982, *History of Ophthalmology*, Volume One, J. P. Wayenborgh Verlag, Bonn, tr. F. C. Blodi.

Locke, J., 1846, *An Essay Concerning Human Understanding*, Thirtieth ed., Thomas Tegg, London, p. 84.

Tychsen, L., 1993, Motion sensitivity and the origins of infantile strabismus, in: *Early Visual Development, Normal and Abnormal* (K. Simons, ed.), Oxford University Press, London, pp. 384–386.

von Noorden, G. K., 1990, *Binocular Vision and Ocular Motility*, Mosby, St. Louis.

von Senden, M., 1960, *Space and Sight*, Free Press, New York, tr. P. Heath.

Wiesel, T. N., 1982, Postnatal development of the visual cortex and the influence of environment, *Nature* **299**:583–591.

2

Functional Organization
of the Visual System

The visual system must convert the pattern of light that falls on the retina into perceptions. This involves a transformation of the visual image in several dimensions. Take, for example, depth perception. There are several cues to depth perception, including disparity, vergence, perspective, shading, texture gradients, interposition, motion parallax, size, and accommodation. For a complete perception, all of these must be analyzed. Where some cues conflict with others (see Kaufman, 1974), the system must resolve the conflicts and come to a decision. Where the cues agree with each other, the system produces a perception of the distance of an object from the subject, its position in relation to other objects nearby, and the three-dimensional shape of the object.

As another example, consider color vision. The most important property of color, for the survival of the species, is not the pleasurable sensations that it gives, but the fact that it helps us recognize objects. The visual system has evolved so that the color of an object remains constant when seen in different sources of illumination, and against different backgrounds. This is known as object color constancy. What is recognized is a property of the object, namely the percentage of each wavelength that is reflected by the object (reflection spectrum). The composition of the wavelengths reaching the eye from the object is the product of the reflection spectrum and the illumination falling on the object: what the visual system does, as Helmholtz put it, is to "discount the source of illumination." This is a complicated calculation, as shown by numerous attempts in the last century to provide a mathematical formula for it.

One could provide a number of other examples from shape perception, pattern perception, and control of eye movements, if space permitted. In all cases, the basic job of the visual system is to recognize objects and their position in space. Sometimes this leads to illusions such as the Ponzo illusion (Fig. 2.1). In this illusion the two cylinders are the same length, but the bottom one appears to be shorter because of the presence of the converging lines. However, this is not so much an illusion as the visual system operating in a sensible way to recognize distance. As another example, the brightness of an object, as well as its color, depends on the background (Fig. 2.2). In this illustration, the ball in

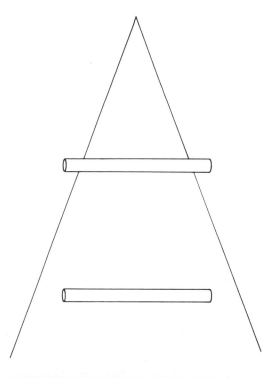

FIG. 2.1. Ponzo illusion. The two cylinders are the same length, but the converging lines make the top cylinder appear longer, because of the effects of perspective.

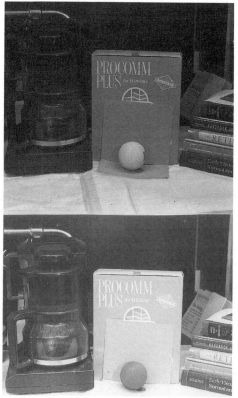

FIG. 2.2. How the brightness of an object depends on the background. Two photographs were taken of a scene, with a light ball in the top scene, and a dark ball in the bottom. Then the whole of the top scene was darkened, so that the amount of light coming from the two balls is identical. Because of contrast with the immediate background, the top ball looks lighter than the bottom one.

the top scene reflects the same amount of light as the ball in the bottom scene, but because the bottom one is seen against a light background, it appears to be darker than the top one. What this chapter is designed to do is to give a broad idea, as far as we know today, of how the visual system is organized to provide these constancies and perceptions.

I. General Anatomical Organization

Initial processing of the image takes place in the retina. The retina projects to four nuclei, with different functions: the lateral geniculate nucleus, for perception of objects; the superior colliculus, for control of eye movements; the pretectum, for control of the pupil; and the suprachiasmatic nucleus, for control of diurnal rhythms and hormonal changes (Fig. 2.3). In most of these areas, and in higher areas of the visual system, there is a topographic organization. That is, the retina maps to the nucleus in an organized fashion. Neighboring parts of the retina project to neighboring parts of the nucleus, so that there is a map of the field of view within the nucleus.

The lateral geniculate nucleus has several layers, and the two eyes project to separate layers. The lateral geniculate projects to primary visual cortex (V1), also known as striate cortex because the input layer can be seen as a stripe without magnification. Primary visual cortex is where the signals from the two eyes come together. There are also projections to the cortex from the superior colliculus through the pulvinar, known as the extrastriate pathway to cortex.

Cortex in general has six layers (I–VI). Signals come in to layer IV. Layer IV

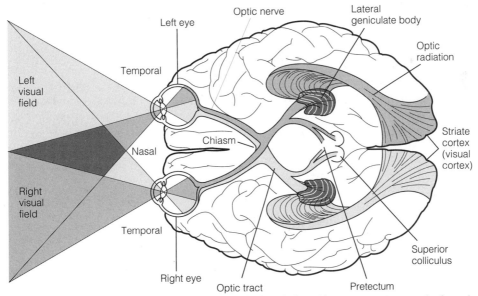

FIG. 2.3. Overall view of the visual system as seen from below. The retina projects to the lateral geniculate body, the superior colliculus, the pretectal area, and the suprachiasmatic nucleus (not shown). The lateral geniculate nucleus projects to the visual cortex. Axons from nasal retina cross in the chiasm, and axons from temporal retina do not. Consequently, the left cortex deals with the right field of view, and vice versa.

projects to layers II and III, which send signals to other areas of cortex. Layers II and III project to layer V, which sends signals back to the superior colliculus. Layers II, III, and V project to layer VI, which sends signals back to the lateral geniculate nucleus. The complete story is far more complicated than this, but these are the predominant projections.

There are a large number of areas in cerebral cortex dealing with vision, at least 32 in macaque monkey (Van Essen *et al.*, 1992) and at least 13 in cat (Rosenquist, 1985). These have been best described in the monkey (Fig. 2.4). The large number of areas, and the even larger number of connections between them—305 at last count in the macaque—is bewildering. Broadly speaking, the areas can be thought of as lying along two pathways. One goes through V1 and secondary visual cortex (V2) and then to temporal cortex and deals primarily with what an object is, that is, its shape, form, and color. The other also goes through V1 and V2 and then to parietal cortex and deals primarily with where an object is and control of eye movements. There is also considerable convergence of signals from different senses in the parietal pathway. The multiplicity of interconnections between areas in the parietal pathway and areas in the temporal pathway shows that this is an oversimplification, but it is a useful one.

Different areas deal with different properties of the visual stimulus. For example, V4 has a lot of cells that respond to color, while V5 (also called MT) has a lot of cells that respond to movement (Zeki, 1978). What specific properties are dealt with in the other 30 or so areas is an active topic of research at the present time. It will be several years before the differences between the various areas are completely characterized.

II. Function in the Retina

The main function of the retina is to convert information about brightness (speaking more correctly, luminance) into information about contrast (Kuffler, 1953). Generally speaking, the visual system is concerned with relative quantities: the luminance of an object in relation to the luminance of objects around it, the long wavelengths coming from an object in relation to medium and short wavelengths, and so on. Many of these relative comparisons are made in the retina. Just about the only function in the visual system that needs luminance information is control of the pupil, and this is dealt with by a special class of cells that goes only to the pretectum.

The retina has five main layers (Fig. 2.5). Light is absorbed by the photoreceptors (rods and cones) which send signals to bipolar cells in the inner nuclear layer, which in turn connect to ganglion cells in the ganglion cell layer. The ganglion cells project to the lateral geniculate nucleus. Then there are two sets of cells which make lateral connections, also with cell bodies in the inner nuclear layer. Horizontal cells make lateral connections between one photoreceptor terminal and another in the outer plexiform layer. Amacrine cells make lateral connections between one bipolar cell terminal and another in the inner plexiform layer. It is these lateral connections that are used to compare signals from light falling on one part of the retina with signals from another part of the retina.

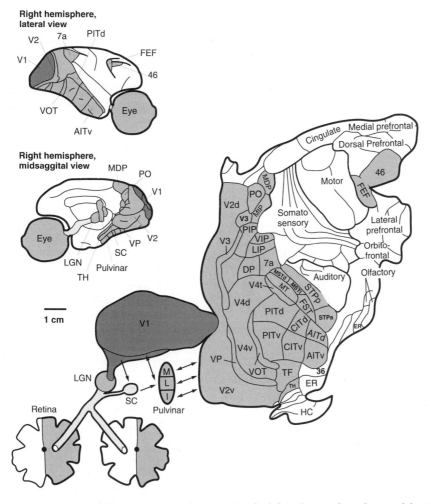

FIG. 2.4. An overview of the macaque visual system. On the left is shown a lateral view of the right cortex (top) and a midsagittal view looking at the medial surface, with the left hemisphere removed (middle). Projections from the retina are summarized at the bottom: the geniculostriate pathway goes from retina to lateral geniculate nucleus (LGN) to V1; the extrastriate pathway goes from retina to superior colliculus (SC) to pulvinar to V2 and other areas. On the right is shown a flattened view of the cortex, with sulci and gyri smoothed out, and with a cut between V1 and V2, which are in reality next to each other, to enable illustration. Visual areas on the temporal pathway dealing with form and color are V4 and inferotemporal areas (PITd, PITv, CITd, CITv, AITd, AITv); visual areas on the parietal pathway dealing with location and eye movements are PO, VIP, LIP, and 7a; MT and MST, which deal with movement, feed into both of these pathways. MIP and VIP receive somatosensory as well as visual input. The function of many areas is not yet defined. Reprinted with permission from Van Essen *et al.*, *Science* 255:419–423. Copyright 1992 American Association for the Advancement of Science.

To understand how these comparisons are made, consider recordings from a bipolar cell, such as the depolarizing cone bipolar cell (Fig. 2.6). The bipolar cell has a "receptive field." The receptive field is defined as including all parts of the retina that affect activity in the bipolar cell. Light falling on photoreceptors that are directly connected to the depolarizing cone bipolar cell will depo-

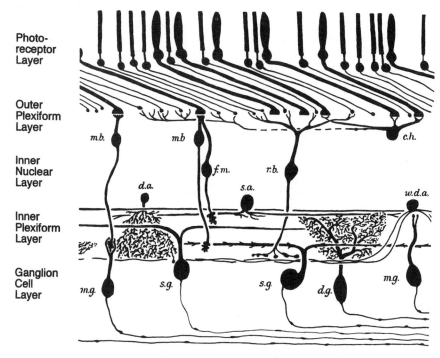

Photo-
receptor
Layer

Outer
Plexiform
Layer

Inner
Nuclear
Layer

Inner
Plexiform
Layer

Ganglion
Cell
Layer

FIG. 2.5. Diagram of various cell types in the macaque monkey and human retinas. Some ganglion cells have small dendritic arborizations (e.g., m.g.) and others have large arborizations (e.g., s.g.). m.b., midget bipolar cell; f.m., flat midget bipolar cell; r.b., rod bipolar cell; c.h., cone horizontal cell; d.a., diffuse amacrine cell; w.d.a., wide diffuse amacrine cell; s.a., stratified amacrine cell; m.g., midget ganglion cell; s.g., stratified ganglion cell; d.g., diffuse ganglion cell. Redrawn with permission from Boycott, B. B., and Dowling, J. E., 1969, Organization of the primate retina: Light microscopy, *Philos. Trans. R. Soc. London* **255**:109–184, Fig. 98 (Royal Society, London).

larize it. Light falling on photoreceptors that are connected indirectly through horizontal cells will oppose or antagonize this influence. Direct connections form the center of the receptive field, and indirect ones the surround. Thus, the bipolar cell will respond to objects falling on the center of its receptive field that are lighter than the background. The hyperpolarizing bipolar cell responds to objects that are darker than the background through a similar process: it is hyperpolarized by light falling in the center of its receptive field and depolarized by light falling on the surround (Werblin and Dowling, 1969).

For color, the first interaction also takes place in horizontal cells, with red-absorbing cones exciting some horizontal cells while green-absorbing cones inhibit them, and blue-absorbing cones exciting other horizontal cells while red- and green-absorbing cones inhibit them (MacNichol and Svaetichin, 1958). These are called red/green and yellow/blue opponent color cells. Cells with the opposite sign of response—excited by green and inhibited by red, or excited by yellow and inhibited by blue—also occur.

Two properties are dealt with at the second stage of processing in the inner plexiform layer. First, a distinction is made between fine detail and movement.

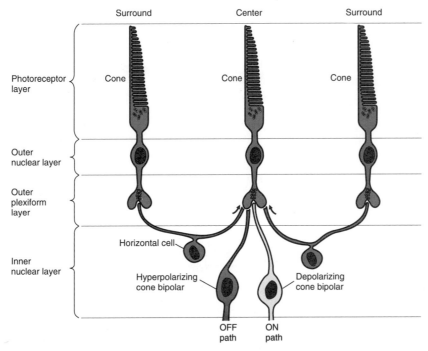

FIG. 2.6. Surround influences in the outer plexiform layer. A cone is connected to the hyper-polarizing cone bipolar cell with a sign-conserving synapse, and to the depolarizing cone bipolar cell with a sign-reversing synapse. At the same time, cones in the surround connect to horizontal cells, which contact the cone in the center and decrease the release of transmitter from it, and consequently antagonize signals going to both types of bipolar cell. Thus, the depolarizing cone bipolar cell is depolarized by light falling on the central cone and its response is reduced when light also falls on the surround. Similarly, the hyperpolarizing cone bipolar cell is hyperpolarized by light falling on the central cone, and its response is also reduced when light also falls on the surround.

Second, the signals from the rods that deal with vision in dim light and the cones that deal with vision in bright light are brought together.

The distinction between fine detail and movement is made in the connections between bipolar cells and ganglion cells (Fig. 2.5). Some ganglion cells receive input from a limited number of bipolar cells and a limited number of photoreceptors (Polyak, 1941). They have small dendritic arborizations, small cell bodies, and give sustained responses. Thus, they have small receptive fields: that is, the area from which photoreceptors feed into them is small, and this is what gives them the ability to analyze fine detail. Examples are the midget ganglion cells in Fig. 2.5. Other ganglion cells receive input from bipolar cells and photoreceptors over a wider area. They have larger dendritic arborizations, larger cell bodies, and give transient responses. Examples are the stratified ganglion cells in Fig. 2.5. It is the transient nature of the response that enables them to respond to movement, even within their receptive field (De Monasterio and Gouras, 1975).

Bipolar cells and ganglion cells connect to each other in the inner plexiform layer with additional local and lateral connections through amacrine cells. The inner plexiform layer is divided into two sublaminae (Famiglietti and Kolb, 1976; see Fig. 2.7). Sublamina b deals with signals for objects brighter than the background: cone bipolar cells that depolarize for such objects connect to ganglion cells that increase their firing rate when a light is turned on and are thus said to have ON responses. Sublamina a deals with signals for objects that are darker than the background: cone bipolar cells that depolarize for such objects connect to ganglion cells that decrease their firing rate when a light is turned on and increase it when a light is turned off and are said to have OFF responses. Signals from the rod photoreceptors feed into this same network

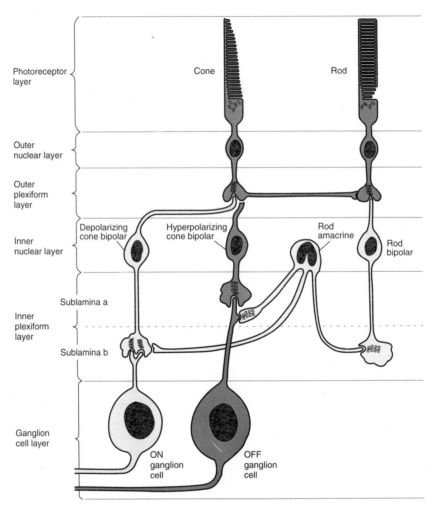

FIG. 2.7. Connections of the inner plexiform layer. Rod amacrine cells and depolarizing cone bipolar cells converge in sublamina b onto ON-center ganglion cells. Hyperpolarizing bipolar cells connect to OFF-center ganglion cells with a sign-conserving synapse, and rod amacrine cells with a sign-reversing synapse in sublamina a. Cells that depolarize in response to light are pale, and cells that hyperpolarize are shaded. Synapses between two pale cells or two shaded cells are sign-conserving, or excitatory; synapses between a shaded cell and a pale cell are sign-reversing, or inhibitory.

through amacrine cells, so that the ganglion cells respond in a similar fashion to both rod and cone signals.

It is the action of these bipolar and ganglion cells that is responsible for our perception of the balls in Fig. 2.2. Depolarizing bipolar cells and ON-center ganglion cells that have the upper ball falling on the center of their receptive fields will fire, signaling that this ball is brighter than the background. Hyperpolarizing bipolar cells and OFF-center ganglion cells that have the lower ball falling on the center of their receptive fields will fire, signaling that the lower ball is darker than the background. Of course, the connections of the bipolar and ganglion cells are fairly short-range, and other cells higher in the system, with long-range connections, will compare the upper ball with the lower ball, but the comparison of an object with its immediately neighboring objects is done in the retina.

The animal models that have been used to study the effects of visual deprivation are cat and monkey. This general picture is similar in cat and monkey, with the exception that the cat has less well-developed color vision. Most of the cones in the cat are green-absorbing: there are a few blue-absorbing cones and no red-absorbing ones, and the percentage of color-coded cells is small. Also, the distinction between fine detail and movement is less pronounced in the cat than in the monkey. The fine detail ganglion cells are called P cells in the monkey, X cells in the cat (Enroth-Cugell and Robson, 1966), and the movement ganglion cells are called M cells in the monkey, Y cells in the cat.

There is another class of ganglion cell found in the cat called W or sluggish cells. This is a heterogeneous class of cells with a variety of different properties (Cleland and Levick, 1974; Stone and Fukuda, 1974). It includes the cells that respond to brightness rather than contrast, and project to the pretectum (sustained ON W cells). The main W cell projection is to superior colliculus, pretectum, and suprachiasmatic nucleus. Some project to the lateral geniculate but the information from most of these is not sent to primary visual cortex from there; therefore, they are not part of the geniculostriate pathway. Although W cells comprise 50% of the ganglion cell population, they have small cell bodies, and are not recorded very frequently in physiological experiments, and therefore less is known about them. There is a class of rarely encountered cells found in the monkey that may correspond to the W cells, but their properties have not received a lot of attention (Schiller and Malpeli, 1977). Partly for this reason, and partly because most of the effects of visual deprivation are found in the geniculostriate pathway, W cells will not get much more mention in this book.

III. Function in the Lateral Geniculate Nucleus

The lateral geniculate nucleus receives signals from the retina and transmits them to the cortex without much processing. Signals from the left and right eyes remain segregated in different layers in the lateral geniculate (Fig. 2.8). In the macaque there are six layers, four dorsal with small cells, thus called the parvocellular layers (P), and two ventral with large cells called magnocellular (M). The fine detail cells project from the retina to the P layers, and the movement cells to the M layers, as reflected in the terminology for these two

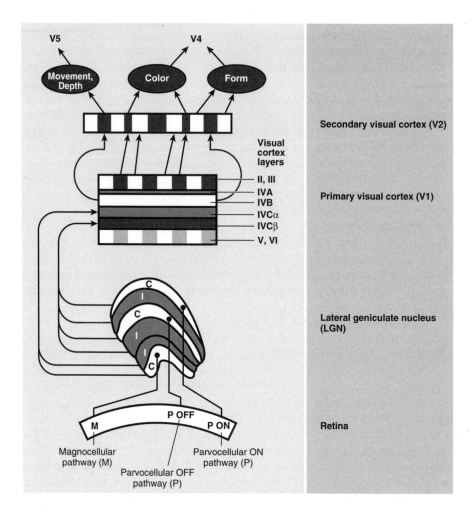

FIG. 2.8. Streams of processing for color, form, and movement between retina and visual cortex. The M pathway projects to the two lower layers in the lateral geniculate nucleus, then to layer IVCα and to layer IVB in primary visual cortex, then to the thick stripes in secondary visual cortex, then to area V5. The P pathway projects to the upper four layers in the lateral geniculate nucleus, with a preponderance of ON-center cells in the upper two layers and OFF-center cells in the middle two layers, then to layer IVCβ. The pathway splits into one dealing with color, which projects from the blobs in layers II and III of primary visual cortex to the thin stripes in secondary visual cortex, then to V4; and one dealing with form, which projects from the interblob areas to the pale stripes in V2 and an area near V4. Input from the contralateral (C) retina is shown. Input from the ipsilateral (I) retina projects to the neighboring layers in the LGN.

groups of cells (see pp. 13–15). Counting from the bottom, layers 1, 4, and 6 receive input from the contralateral eye, and layers 2, 3, and 5 from the ipsilateral eye.

The properties of cells in the lateral geniculate are very like those of the cells in the retina that project to them (Wiesel and Hubel, 1966). There are cells that are excited by light in the center of their receptive field, and inhibited by light in the surrounding area—ON-center cells, just as in the retina. There are cells whose activity is reduced by light in the center, and increased by light in the surround—OFF-center cells. There are red/green and yellow/blue color-coded cells. There does not seem to be much convergence from different cell types in the retina onto single cells in the lateral geniculate. The main difference between LGN and retinal cells that has been noted is that LGN cells give less response to white light illuminating the whole receptive field uniformly. This occurs because there are additional inhibitory interneurons in the lateral geniculate, so that antagonism from the surround of the receptive field of a cell more closely balances the center.

The lateral geniculate receives input from the various modulatory pathways located in the brain stem: noradrenaline input from the locus coeruleus, serotonin input from the raphe nuclei, and acetylcholine input from the parabrachial region (Sherman and Koch, 1986). It also receives some input from the eye movement system. These inputs modulate signals reaching the cortex, by affecting attention, and also by directly inhibiting signals while saccadic eye movements are being made. Essentially, the function of the lateral geniculate nucleus is to gate signals going from the retina to the cortex, rather than to process them.

IV. Function in the Visual Cortex

The visual cortex is the place where objects in and out of their visual context are analyzed in detail. For the analysis of form, there are cells responding to edges and corners of objects. For the analysis of movement, there are cells responding to direction of movement, and direction of movement in relation to the background. For the analysis of color, there are cells responding to wavelengths coming from an object in relation to wavelengths coming from objects nearby, and an average of wavelengths from objects in other parts of the field of view.

To a certain extent, form, color, movement, and depth are dealt with by separate groups of cells. Because of this, layer IV, which is the input layer for the cortex, is more complicated in visual cortex than in any other area of cortex (Fig. 2.8). It is divided into sublayers IVA, IVB, IVCα, and IVCβ. Projections from the movement cells in the magnocellular layers of the lateral geniculate come into layer IVCα, which projects to layer IVB. Layer IVB projects to secondary visual cortex (V2), and is therefore an output layer rather than an input layer. The movement cells in V2 project to an area of visual cortex called V5 or MT, which deals specifically with movement (Zeki, 1978), and from there to an area called MST, which also deals with movement.

The cells in the parvocellular layers of the lateral geniculate, dealing with color and fine detail, project to layers IVCβ and IVA (Fig. 2.8). These signals are analyzed further in other layers of primary visual cortex. If one makes a horizontal section through primary visual cortex in layers III and II, and stains it for cytochrome oxidase, the mitochondrial enzyme that is found in areas of high metabolic activity, one finds patches of stain known as blobs. Color-coded cells are concentrated in the blobs, while the cells in the areas between the blobs respond to the orientation of an edge (Livingstone and Hubel, 1984).

In secondary visual cortex (V2), cells dealing with color, form, and movement are also kept separate. If one stains V2 with cytochrome oxidase, and makes a horizontal section, one finds three sets of stripes—thick stripes, thin stripes, and pale stripes (Livingstone and Hubel, 1987). The color-coded cells in the blobs project to the thin stripes. The cells specific for orientation between the blobs project to the pale stripes. The cells specific for movement in layer IVB project to the thick stripes. The thin stripes then project to an area called V4, which deals particularly with color. The thick stripes are the ones that project to V5 and MST.

Visual cortex is the first location in which signals from the two eyes converge onto a single cell. Signals in layer IV are kept largely separate in the adult, but the monocular cells in layer IV converge onto binocular cells in layers II, III, V, and VI. This is a statistical matter rather than an absolute matter—there are some binocular cells in layer IV and some monocular cells in layers II, III, V, and VI—but the tendency is clear. Consequently, visual cortex is the first location where one finds cells sensitive to disparity—that is, cells responding to objects nearer than the point of fixation, and cells responding to objects farther than the point of fixation (Poggio *et al.*, 1988). Disparity-sensitive cells are concentrated in the same stripes as movement cells in V2 (Hubel and Livingstone, 1987), but their anatomical location in V1 remains to be clarified.

V. The Columnar Organization of Cortex

Cells located above and below each other in the cortex tend to have similar properties. This is true in all parts of cortex, and was first noticed in the somatosensory cortex (Mountcastle, 1957), and then in the visual cortex of the cat (Hubel and Wiesel, 1962). Consequently, the cortex is said to be organized into columns. The similar properties of cells in a column are most likely related to the arrangement of anatomical connections, which run primarily in a vertical direction.

In the monkey, there are columns for ocular dominance, color, and orientation of edges (Livingstone and Hubel, 1984). While cells in layers II, III, V, and VI tend to be binocular, they also tend to be dominated by one eye. A cell dominated by the left eye in layer II will tend to lie above endings from the left eye in layer IV, a cell dominated by the right eye in layer VI will tend to be below endings from the right eye in layer IV, and so on. Color-coded cells in layer V or VI tend to lie under the blobs in layers III and II. When it comes to orientation, there are cells specific for vertical edges, cells specific for horizontal edges, and cells specific for a variety of orientations in between. Again, the cells specific for vertical edges in layers V and VI tend to lie below the cells specific for vertical edges in layers II and III.

Every point in the field of view has to be analyzed for color and orientation for each eye, so that the sets of columns overlap each other (Fig. 2.9). A system of ocular dominance columns is superimposed on a system of orientation columns, with the blobs for color stuck in. Thus, there is a module for each part of the field of view, called a hypercolumn, in which an analysis of the various features of the stimulus takes place. Of course, biology is not as neatly rectangu-

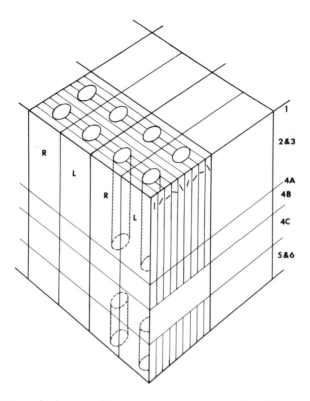

FIG. 2.9. Organization of columns and layers in macaque striate cortex. Columns for left and right eyes (L and R) overlap with columns for various orientations. Pegs for the columns dealing with color are interspersed into the orientation system. Note that orientation is missing from the pegs, and from layer IVCβ, where the fine detail lateral geniculate afferents come in. Moreover, the pegs for color do not go through layers IVB and IVCα, which deal with movement. Reprinted with permission from Livingstone and Hubel (1984).

lar as shown in Fig. 2.9, but the general principle is illustrated. The movement system, in area 17 of primate, is an exception to the general rule of columnar processing: signals come in to layer IVCα, project to layer IVB, then project out of primary visual cortex. However, this is the only known exception: in all other parts of cortex, processing is columnar. Organization in the cat primary visual cortex is the same, except that color cells are absent (color-coded cells are mostly in the W cell projection, in the extrastriate pathway). Thus, there are just two sets of overlapping columns, for orientation and ocular dominance.

The visual properties dealt with in columns in V2 are not too different from the columnar properties of V1. As mentioned above, the thin stripes of cytochrome oxidase staining deal with color coding, the pale stripes deal with orientation and form, and the thick stripes deal with movement.

Beyond V2, the parameters of the stimulus dealt with in columns are less clear. Obviously the parameters will change with the visual area, since different visual areas deal with different properties of the stimulus. In V4, there are probably columns for red, columns for green, and columns for blue (Zeki, 1977). In V5, there are columns for direction of movement (Albright et al.,

1984), and for movement of objects in relation to the background as opposed to movement of the whole field of view (Born and Tootell, 1992). The physiological details remain to be worked out in areas V4 and V5 and are completely unknown in the other 30 areas of visual cortex, but every anatomical experiment that has been done shows punctate projections from one area to another, strongly suggesting the existence of columns everywhere.

VI. Parallel Processing within the Visual System

It should be clear by now that different features of the stimulus are dealt with in parallel with each other in the visual system. Signals for objects brighter than the background and signals for objects darker than the background are kept separate through four levels of processing—bipolar cell, ganglion cell, lateral geniculate cell, and first stage within V1—before being combined to analyze orientation and direction of movement, independent of contrast (Fig. 2.8). Signals for color and signals for movement are kept separate through at least five levels of processing: ganglion cell, lateral geniculate, V1, V2, and V4/V5. Signals for color and signals for form are kept separate through at least three levels of processing: V1, V2, and V4 (the area for processing of form in the macaque at the level of V4 is not well identified, but it seems likely from deficits found in humans that there are separate areas for color and form at this level).

Very likely, parallel processing will continue to be found, as higher levels of cortex are analyzed. Depth perception remains to be worked out. How the various cues to depth perception are analyzed and brought together is largely unknown. Cells sensitive for disparity are found in V1 and in the thick stripes of V2 and in V3. Whether there are separate columns for near and far cells at any of these stages is not known. However the details may work out, it seems extremely likely that depth perception will be analyzed by columns in a parallel fashion, because there are a variety of cues that have to be evaluated and then combined.

VII. Hierarchical Processing within the Visual System

What happens to the signals, as they get transmitted within these parallel pathways, and are processed along the way? The first work to be done came from Hubel and Wiesel (1962) and concerned the analysis of form in the cat. They recorded from single cells in the visual cortex with a microelectrode in anesthetized paralyzed animals. Interestingly, the cells responded much more vigorously to bars and edges, particularly moving ones, than to lights turned on and off. There were cells that responded to orientation with separate cells for lines brighter than the background and for lines darker than the background. They called these *simple cells*, because the properties could be explained simply by input from a series of lateral geniculate cells lined up along the axis of the orientation (Fig. 2.10). They also found cells that respond to orientation independent of contrast, and called those *complex cells*, and proposed that

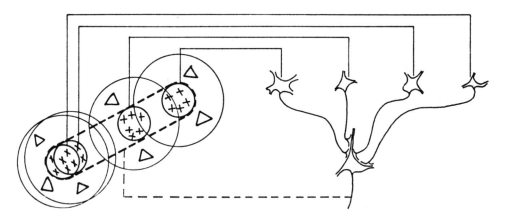

FIG. 2.10. Scheme for producing simple cells from lateral geniculate input to the cortex. Four lateral geniculate cells with ON centers, lined up along a line, make excitatory connections with a cell in the cortex. The cortical cell will then respond to a line oriented along the 2 o'clock/8 o'clock axis. Reprinted with permission from Hubel and Wiesel (1962).

they receive input from simple cells. Some cells responded to short bars, because of inhibitory influences, and were called *hypercomplex*, while the simple and complex cells responded to long ones. Subsequent investigators have found that the complex cells actually receive direct input from the lateral geniculate (see Stone, 1983), but the basic idea of a hierarchical organization in these cell types is nonetheless probably true.

Clearer evidence for a hierarchy of cell types comes from the color system (Daw, 1984). Photoreceptors converge onto the "opponent color cells" referred to on p. 12 (see Fig. 2.11). Within the color system, bipolar cells, ganglion cells, lateral geniculate cells, and cells within layer IVCβ of the cortex are all opponent color cells. At the next stage, in the blobs in V1, opponent color cells converge to form double opponent cells. These are cells that are opponent for color and also for space so that they respond to color contrasts and some spatial contrasts, but not to uniform illumination (see caption of Fig. 2.11). The response of a red/green double opponent cell to a gray spot in a green surround is the same as its response to a red spot in a gray surround: gray will activate both red and green receptors, with responses that will cancel each other, while red in the center and green in the surround will both excite the cell. Since a gray spot in a green surround appears reddish (this is called simultaneous color contrast), double opponent cells explain the phenomenon of simultaneous color contrast (Daw, 1967).

Simultaneous color contrast is a local phenomenon, whereas object color constancy involves comparisons over a large part of the field of view. Cells in V1 have small receptive fields, whereas cells in V4 have large ones. Cells in V4 are affected by an average of the wavelengths coming from objects in a wide area of the field of view. Thus, it seems likely that the double opponent cells in V1 converge onto cells in V2, and these converge again onto cells in V4 to give object color constancy (Zeki, 1983).

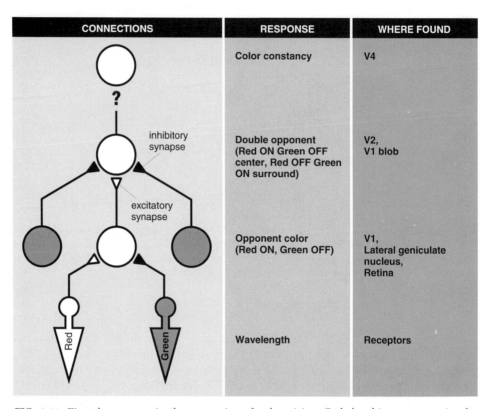

CONNECTIONS	RESPONSE	WHERE FOUND
	Color constancy	V4
inhibitory synapse	Double opponent (Red ON Green OFF center, Red OFF Green ON surround)	V2, V1 blob
excitatory synapse	Opponent color (Red ON, Green OFF)	V1, Lateral geniculate nucleus, Retina
Red Green	Wavelength	Receptors

FIG. 2.11. First three stages in the processing of color vision. Red-absorbing cones excite the bipolar cells, and green cones inhibit them, to produce bipolar cells, ganglion cells, lateral geniculate cells, and cells in layer IVCβ that give an ON response to red and an OFF response to green. Red ON/green OFF cells in the center of the receptive field excite the double opponent cell, and red ON/green OFF cells in the surround inhibit it. This produces a cell that has an ON response to red, an OFF response to green in the center, and an OFF response to red, ON response to green in the surround, because the sign of the response is reversed in the surround by the inhibitory synapse. Double opponent cells do not respond to uniform illumination (in the example illustrated, excitation from red in the center will be canceled by inhibition from red in the periphery, and excitation from green in the periphery will be canceled by inhibition from green in the center). Double opponent cells also do not respond to white light, because the input from the red receptors will be canceled by the input from the green receptors. The synaptic organization between V1, V2, and V4 is not known, but the cells in V4 give a response that corresponds to object color constancy. Open triangles represent excitatory synapses, closed triangles inhibitory synapses.

Evidence for a hierarchy of cell types is also clear in the movement system (Fig. 2.12). Cells in the magnocellular pathway in the retina and the lateral geniculate respond to movement. In primary visual cortex, one finds cells that respond to *direction* of movement, because of lateral inhibitory connections. In V5, there are cells that respond to movement of the complete object, as opposed to movement of the individual contours of the object (Movshon et al., 1985). There are also cells that respond to movement of an object in relation to the background, rather than movement of the object itself (Tanaka et al., 1986; see Fig. 2.13).

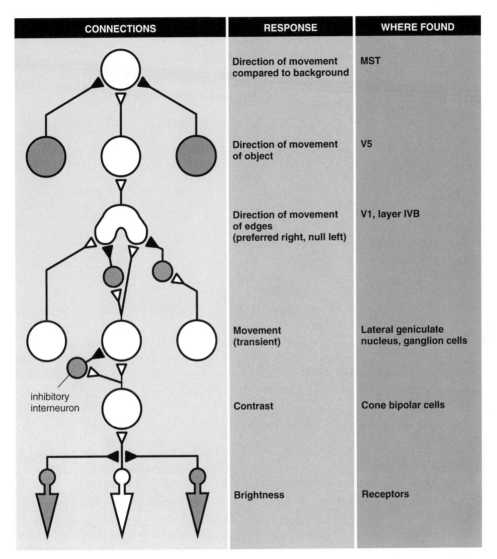

CONNECTIONS	RESPONSE	WHERE FOUND
	Direction of movement compared to background	MST
	Direction of movement of object	V5
	Direction of movement of edges (preferred right, null left)	V1, layer IVB
	Movement (transient)	Lateral geniculate nucleus, ganglion cells
inhibitory interneuron	Contrast	Cone bipolar cells
	Brightness	Receptors

FIG. 2.12. First five stages in the processing of movement information. Receptors respond to brightness and bipolar cells to contrast. Some circuit, perhaps a local inhibitory circuit, makes the response of the movement ganglion cells transient, and consequently the response of the movement lateral geniculate cells that follow them. Lateral inhibitory connections within the visual cortex reduce the response in one direction, to produce direction-selective cells. The synaptic circuitry that produces a cell specific for movement of the object, as opposed to movement of the contours within the object, is not known, and is therefore left out. Presumably direction of movement of the object in relation to its background is produced by excitatory connections from the direction-selective cells that are processing the object, and inhibitory connections from the direction-selective cells that are processing the background. Open triangles represent excitatory synapses, closed triangles inhibitory synapses.

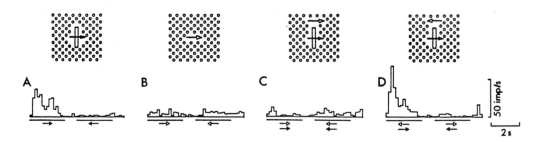

FIG. 2.13. Cell that responds to movement of an object against its background. (A) Response to movement of bar. (B) Response to movement of background. (C) Response to movement of bar and background together in the same direction. (D) Response to movement of bar and background in opposite directions. Notice that movement of the bar against the background gives the largest response, and movement of the bar with the background gives little response. Reprinted with permission from Tanaka *et al.* (1986).

VIII. Summary

Hopefully this brief summary will give an idea of how the visual system is organized. There are streams of cells dealing with broad aspects of the scene, with details analyzed in parallel to each other within the streams.

In the color stream, red/green, yellow/blue, and black/white aspects are processed in parallel with each other. As one goes up the system, a comparison is first made between the long, medium, and short bands of wavelengths coming from a small area in the field of view. This is then compared to the area in the immediate surround, and then to a large part of the field of view to give a perception of object color constancy.

In the form stream, objects lighter than the background and objects darker than the background are first distinguished. The orientation of edges and lines is analyzed, then the length of segments of the edges and lines.

In the movement stream, the response is made transient within the retina, to enable movement to be detected. Lateral inhibitory connections operate on signals from the brighter-than-background pathway and on signals from the darker-than-background pathway, to give direction of movement, then these are brought together to give a perception of direction of movement independent of contrast. Next, signals for the direction of movement of contours are combined to give the direction of movement of the whole object. Then the direction of movement of the object in relation to the background is distinguished from direction of movement of the object by itself.

In the depth system, disparity is detected immediately after signals from the two eyes come together in the cortex. There are cells specific for objects nearer than the fixation point, and cells specific for objects farther away than the fixation point. Disparity is actually a relative phenomenon, like brightness and color, but cells specific for relative disparity have not yet been described, and how disparity is related to other cues about depth perception is unknown.

The concentration on streams of processing in this description is an oversimplification. Edges can be detected between two colored objects of equal luminance, showing that color signals enter the form pathway. Although some displays of stereopsis fail when one object is seen in relation to another of equal luminance, other displays succeed. Consequently, perceptual experiments suggest that there must be connections between the various streams, and the anatomy proves that there are. However, the division of the visual system into streams of processing is a useful concept for understanding the overall organization.

References

Albright, T. D., Desimone, R., and Gross, C. G., 1984, Columnar organization of directionally selective cells in visual area MT of the macaque, *J. Neurophysiol.* **51**:16–31.

Born, R. T., and Tootell, R. B. H., 1992, Segregation of global and local motion processing in primate middle temporal visual area, *Nature* **357**:497–499.

Boycott, B. B., and Dowling, J. E., 1969, Organization of the primate retina: Light microscopy, *Philos. Trans. R. Soc. London Ser. B.* **255**:109–184.

Cleland, B. G., and Levick, W. R., 1974, Properties of rarely encountered types of ganglion cells in the cat's retina and an overall classification, *J. Physiol. (London)* **240**:457–492.

Daw, N. W., 1967, Goldfish retina: Organization for simultaneous color contrast, *Science* **158**:942–944.

Daw, N. W., 1984, The psychology and physiology of colour vision, *Trends Neurosci.* **7**:330–336.

De Monasterio, F. M., and Gouras, P., 1975, Functional properties of ganglion cells of the rhesus monkey retina, *J. Physiol. (London)* **251**:167–195.

Enroth-Cugell, C., and Robson, J. G., 1966, The contrast sensitivity of retinal ganglion cells of the cat, *J. Physiol. (London)* **187**:517–552.

Famiglietti, E. V., and Kolb, H., 1976, Structural basis for ON- and OFF-center responses in retinal ganglion cells, *Science* **194**:193–195.

Hubel, D. H., and Livingstone, M. S., 1987, Segregation of form, color, and stereopsis in primate area 18, *J. Neurosci.* **7**:3378–3415.

Hubel, D. H., and Wiesel, T. N., 1962, Receptive fields, binocular interaction and functional architecture in cat's visual cortex, *J. Physiol. (London)* **160**:106–154.

Kaufman, L., 1974, *Sight and Mind*, Oxford University Press, London.

Kuffler, S. W., 1953, Discharge patterns and functional organization of mammalian retina, *J. Neurophysiol.* **16**:37–68.

Livingstone, M. S., and Hubel, D. H., 1984, Anatomy and physiology of a color system in the primate visual cortex, *J. Neurosci.* **4**:309–356.

Livingstone, M. S., and Hubel, D. H., 1987, Connections between layer 4B of area 17 and thick cytochrome oxidase stripes of area 18 in the squirrel monkey, *J. Neurosci.* **7**:3371–3377.

MacNichol, E. F., and Svaetichin, G., 1958, Electric responses from the isolated retinas of fishes, *Am. J. Ophthalmol.* **46**:26–46.

Mountcastle, V. B., 1957, Modality and topographic properties of single neurons of cat's somatic sensory cortex, *J. Neurophysiol.* **20**:408–434.

Movshon, J. A., Adelson, E. H., Gizzi, M. S., and Newsome, W. T., 1985, The analysis of moving visual patterns, in: *Pattern Recognition Mechanisms* (C. Chaga, R. Gattass, and C. Gross, eds.), Pontifical Academy of Sciences, Vatican City, pp. 117–151.

Poggio, G. F., Gonzalez, F., and Krause, F., 1988, Stereoscopic mechanisms in monkey visual cortex: Binocular correlation and disparity selectivity, *J. Neurosci.* **8**:4531–4550.

Polyak, S. L., 1941, *The Retina*, University of Chicago Press, Chicago.

Rosenquist, A., 1985, Connections of visual cortical areas in the cat, in: *Cerebral Cortex* (A. Peters and E. G. Jones, eds.), Plenum Press, New York, pp. 81–117.

Schiller, P. H., and Malpeli, J. G., 1977, Properties and tectal projections of monkey ganglion cells, *J. Neurophysiol.* **40**:428–445.

Sherman, S. M., and Koch, C., 1986, The control of retinogeniculate transmission in the mammalian lateral geniculate nucleus, *Exp. Brain Res.* **63**:1–20.

Stone, J., 1983, *Parallel Processing in the Visual System*, Plenum Press, New York.

Stone, J., and Fukuda, Y., 1974, Properties of cat retinal ganglion cells: A comparison of W-cells with X- and Y-cells, *J. Neurophysiol.* **37:**722–748.

Tanaka, K., Hikosaka, K., Saito, H. E., Yukie, M., Fukada, Y., and Iwai, E., 1986, Analysis of local and wide-field movements in the superior temporal visual areas of the macaque monkey, *J. Neurosci.* **6:**134–144.

Van Essen, D. C., Anderson, C. H., and Felleman, D. J., 1992, Information processing in the primate visual system: An integrated systems perspective, *Science* **255:**419–423.

Werblin, F. S., and Dowling, J. E., 1969, Organization of the retina of the mudpuppy, Necturus maculosus. II. Intracellular recording, *J. Neurophysiol.* **32:**339–355.

Wiesel, T. N., and Hubel, D. H., 1966, Spatial and chromatic interactions in the lateral geniculate body of the rhesus monkey, *J. Neurophysiol.* **29:**1115–1156.

Zeki, S. M., 1977, Colour coding in the superior temporal sulcus of the rhesus monkey visual cortex, *Proc. R. Soc. London B Ser.* **197:**195–223.

Zeki, S. M., 1978, Uniformity and diversity of structure and function in rhesus monkey prestriate visual cortex, *J. Physiol. (London)* **277:**273–290.

Zeki, S. M., 1983, Colour coding in the cerebral cortex: The reaction of cells in monkey visual cortex to wavelengths and colours, *Neuroscience* **9:**741–765.

Normal Development

3

Development of Visual Capabilities

Infants can presumably see at birth. They can imitate mouth opening, as opposed to tongue protrusion, within a few hours of birth (Salapatek and Cohen, 1987). While they may not discriminate their mother's face reliably from a stranger's, unless voice is present, they do look at their mother for longer than the stranger. They may not look their mother in the eye until 2 months of age, but this is because they are inspecting external features of the face, such as the chin and hairline, rather than internal features, such as the eyes. All of this shows a substantial amount of visual perception at birth, and some control of eye movements. What develops after birth is a refinement of these properties.

The development of visual capabilities over the first few months is a coordinated matter, involving both sensory and motor aspects. Indeed, looking at objects is very much a sensory-motor activity. To put it briefly, the adult visual system can be thought of as three systems. We notice objects in the peripheral part of the field of view, and move the eyes with a saccadic movement to look at them if they demand attention. We converge the eyes to look at nearby objects, and diverge them to look at objects far away, so that the images in the two eyes can be fused into a single perception. Then we use the central part of the field of view to inspect objects and analyze their form, color, and distance in relation to other objects. Even the inspection of an object involves some eye movements, because the perception of images that remain stationary on the retina fades away. To avoid this, the eyes drift slowly across the object, interspersed with small jerks called microsaccades. Fixation of one's gaze on an object is therefore an active process rather than a passive one.

Thus, improvement of the ability to see fine detail in an object depends on the ability to keep one's eyes tightly fixated on it. Likewise, improvement in binocular function goes hand in hand with the ability to converge or diverge one's eyes to look at the object. There is a cycle in the system: better sensory capability leading to more accurate eye movements leading to better sensory capability and so on.

Before dealing with the development of responses to visual stimuli, we need to ask: is the image on the infant retina a clear one? Is the limiting step in analysis of the image the clarity of the image, or the processing within the nervous system? The infant retina can be seen clearly with an ophthalmoscope.

There do not appear to be any optical aberrations in the cornea or lens that would degrade the image substantially. The surfaces of the lens and cornea grow along with the eye, so that objects remain in focus for most children (Howland, 1993). Most infants have astigmatism—a cylindrical component to the focusing of the image on the retina—so that lines along one axis are in focus, while lines along the perpendicular axis are not. However, this is probably too small in most cases to have perceptual consequences.

Infants have some ability to accommodate their focus to objects at different distances at 2 weeks of age, and this ability increases during the first 3 months of age (Banks, 1980). There are several cues that adults use to control accommodation, e.g., blur, vergence, chromatic aberration, and disparity (see Glossary). We do not know which ones are used by young infants, except that disparity cannot be used soon after birth, since the neuronal detection of disparity does not develop until later. The need for infants to accommodate is much less than in adults, because infants have a greater depth of focus, as a result of a smaller pupil diameter. Also, their acuity is one-tenth that of adults, so that they cannot detect whether an object is in or out of focus as well as can an adult. The fact that they do not make large accommodative efforts is related to lack of need, as much as lack of ability.

Thus, with the exception of some astigmatism, the image that falls on the infant retina is a clear one, and the infant can make adjustments for objects at different distances. Therefore, as vision develops, it is not the optics of the eyeball that develop, as much as the properties of the photoreceptors, the retina, and the central visual system.

I. Methods for Studying Infant Vision

The history of the investigation of infant vision is a history of techniques as much as a history of discoveries. Infants cannot talk, and are often inattentive. Two types of response have been monitored: gross electrophysiological responses, such as the visual evoked potential and the electroretinogram; and eye movement responses, such as fixation on an object of interest, and optokinetic nystagmus. As pointed out above, sensory and motor capabilities develop in tandem, so that an infant may not look at an object even though he/she sees it. In the case of electrophysiological responses, gross measurements represent the average of the firing of all of the neurons involved. As a result, all measurements give a lower limit for the capability of the infant, and the actual capability may be higher. It is a tribute to the determination of the investigators that results from the various techniques agree with each other, and that modeling sometimes shows that the results are close to a theoretical limit, in which case the actual capability has been revealed.

In studying infant vision, psychologists have been concerned with a quantitative or psychophysical measurement of what infants see. As an example, consider acuity. This is measured in the ophthalmologist's office by looking at letters of the alphabet. If a person sees a letter at 20 feet that a normal person could see at 40 feet, they are said to have an acuity of 20/40 (Snellen acuity). Infants cannot read letters, so a grating is presented instead, and some technique is used to detect whether the infant can discriminate the grating from a uniform gray stimulus. Then one varies the spatial frequency of the grating, which is measured in cycles per degree (the number of lines in the grating that subtend 1° as seen by the observer). 20/20 vision corresponds to 30 cycles/degree.

The technique most frequently used is called the forced-choice preferential looking procedure (FPL). This depends on the propensity of infants to look at an "interesting" display more often than a less interesting display. An infant is seated looking at two displays with a peephole between them (Teller, 1977). An observer, who does not know which display is which, decides whether the infant looks more at the left display or the right display (Fig. 3.1). The position of the "interesting" display is changed to left or right in a random order. A positive result (the records from the observer show that the infant is looking at the "interesting" display more often than the other more than 75% of the time)

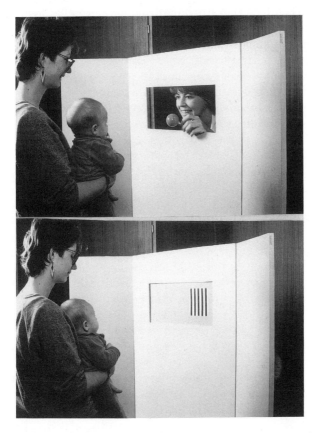

FIG. 3.1. The forced-choice preferential looking procedure. The observer attracts the infant's attention toward the opening in the screen (top). Then the test cards are presented, and the observer monitors the infant's behavior through a central peephole, marked in the figure by an arrow (bottom). Reprinted with kind permission from Katz, B., and Sireteanu, R., 1990, The Teller acuity card test: A useful method for the clinical routine? *Clin. Vision Sci.* **5:**307–323. Copyright 1990, Elsevier Science, Ltd., The Boulevard, Langford Lane, Kidlington OX5 1GB, UK.

is significant, but a negative result could be related to inattentiveness on the part of the infant or inexperience on the part of the observer rather than failure of the infant to discriminate the displays.

Also used quite frequently is the visual evoked potential (VEP). This is a potential recorded from the scalp of the infant by electrodes placed over the visual cortex. The infant does not have to be paying attention for this technique to work, but does need to fixate and accommodate, and the stimulus has to be one that will activate enough neurons in the cortex in synchrony with each other that their combined activity shows up as an electrical change on the surface. Some investigators have been quite ingenious in devising stimuli that get good results with this technique.

The electroretinogram (ERG) is a potential recorded between the cornea and the skin that represents the summed activity of cells in the retina. Thus, it can only be used to study properties of the retina, such as dark adaptation (see below). Optokinetic nystagmus (OKN) is an oscillation of the eyes produced when looking at a stimulus slowly moving in one direction. The eyes follow the stimulus, then flick back in the reverse direction with a saccade-like movement. OKN is believed to be primarily a subcortical phenomenon, and needs a large stimulus covering a substantial amount of the visual field. Both of these procedures are therefore of limited utility.

All of these techniques have been primarily useful in testing discriminative ability, and demonstrating changes in properties that can be quantified, such as acuity and stereopsis. When it comes to what the infant sees, we are still often at a loss. We can study wavelength discrimination, but not very much about color vision. If, as seems likely, a child can recognize the faces of its mother and father long before it can say "mama" and "dada," we can only guess at many aspects of infant visual perception.

II. Development of Monocular Vision

In spite of all of the problems with the techniques listed above, many visual properties have been studied successfully. For monocular vision, this includes acuity, contrast sensitivity, increment thresholds, adaptation, spectral sensitivity, perception of direction and orientation, and vernier acuity (see Glossary).

A. Acuity

This property is usually studied with a grating of black and white lines. When FPL is used, the infant is presented with a choice of a grating (the "interesting" stimulus) or a uniform stimulus of the same luminance (see stimuli in Fig. 3.1). The limit of acuity is represented by the finest grating that can be distinguished reliably from the uniform stimulus. When the VEP is measured, the most successful stimulus is a "sweep" stimulus (Norcia and Tyler, 1985). The contrast of the grating is reversed at 12 cycles/sec, and the spatial frequency is incremented (swept) every 0.5 sec, so that results from several spatial frequencies can be recorded in a short period of time.

There are some differences between the numbers generated by different experimenters and different techniques, but the agreement is actually quite remarkable. There is a large improvement found in all cases between birth and 6 months of age, from about 1 cycle/degree (20/600) to about 25 cycles/degree (20/24), and some further improvement after that (Fig. 3.2).

A large part of the development of acuity can be explained by changes that occur in the retina in the size, shape, and distribution of photoreceptors, and in the optics of the eye (Banks and Bennett, 1988). The eye is shorter in the newborn, and the pupil is smaller; consequently, the image on the retina falls on a smaller area. The photoreceptors—and here we are concerned with the

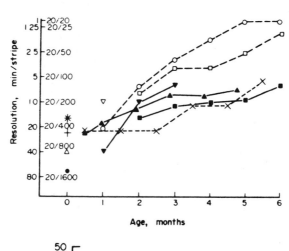

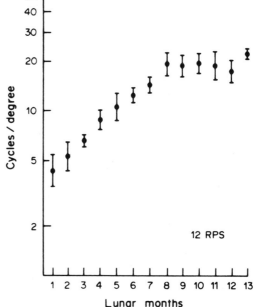

FIG. 3.2. Improvement of acuity with age. Shown on the top is a compendium of results from different authors, using different techniques. Shown on the bottom are measurements using the "sweep" technique, from Norcia and Tyler (1985, Fig. 7). Top reprinted with kind permission from Dobson, V., and Teller, D. Y., 1978, Visual acuity in human infants: A review and comparison of behavioral and electrophysiological techniques, *Vision Res.* **18:**1469–1483. Copyright 1978, Elsevier Science, Ltd., The Boulevard, Langford Lane, Kidlington OX5 1GB, UK. Right reprinted with kind permission from Norcia, A. M., and Tyler, C. W., 1985, Spatial frequency sweep VEP: Visual acuity during the first year of life, *Vision Res.* **25:**1399–1408. Copyright 1985, Elsevier Science, Ltd., The Boulevard, Langford Lane, Kidlington OX5 1GB, UK.

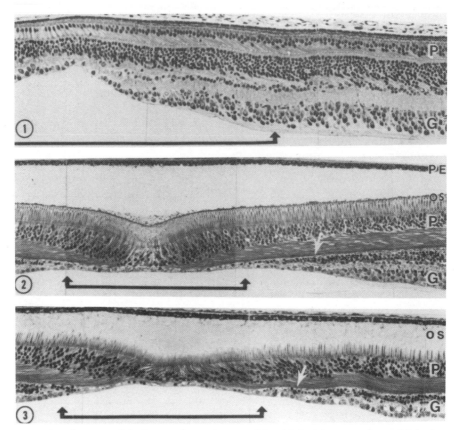

FIG. 3.3. Development of the human fovea. Ages are (1) at birth, (2) 45 months, and (3) 72 years. Note that the rod-free area, marked by black arrows, becomes smaller; and the cone outer segments in the fovea become narrower and longer. Reprinted with kind permission from Yuodelis, C., and Hendrickson, A., 1986, A qualitative and quantitative analysis of the human fovea during development, *Vision Res.* **26:**847–855. Copyright 1986, Elsevier Science, Ltd., The Boulevard, Langford Lane, Kidlington OX5 1GB, UK.

cone photoreceptors in the fovea, which is the region of highest acuity—are wider in the newborn (more than 6 μm, compared to 1.9 μm in the adult—see Fig. 3.3), so that they are spaced farther apart (Yuodelis and Hendrickson, 1986). The outer segment of each individual photoreceptor is shorter, and absorbs less light. These factors combine to predict a substantial improvement in acuity with age, as the percentage of the light falling on the photoreceptor that is absorbed is increased, and the width of an object that is covered by a single photoreceptor is reduced. However, they do not predict it all. Whereas acuity in the adult is close to the theoretical limit imposed by the properties of the eye and its photoreceptors, acuity in the newborn is not. There must be, in addition, some factors in the neural networks beyond the photoreceptors that restrict newborn acuity to a value less than the theoretical limit. These factors will be discussed in Chapter 5.

B. Contrast Sensitivity

Sensitivity to contrast is a property that has been used to analyze several different aspects of the visual system. How sensitivity to contrast varies with spatial frequency can be seen in a display of sinusoidal stripes which vary in spatial frequency along one axis, and in contrast along the orthogonal axis (Fig. 3.4). At high spatial frequencies, the stripes cannot be seen, no matter how high the contrast. At medium spatial frequencies, quite low contrasts can be seen— less than 1% of the overall luminance in adults. At low spatial frequencies, a larger contrast is needed for visibility than at medium spatial frequencies (this is called low-frequency falloff).

In experiments with infants, the subject is presented with a grating of uniform spatial frequency and contrast, and observed to see if the stripes are being detected. The lowest contrast that can be seen at each spatial frequency is recorded, and a curve is generated (Fig. 3.5). This curve is an accurate measurement of the positions where the stripes become invisible in Fig. 3.4, which can be seen and traced approximately by hand. Needless to say, the actual experimental procedure is time-consuming and results are slow to develop, particularly when working with infants.

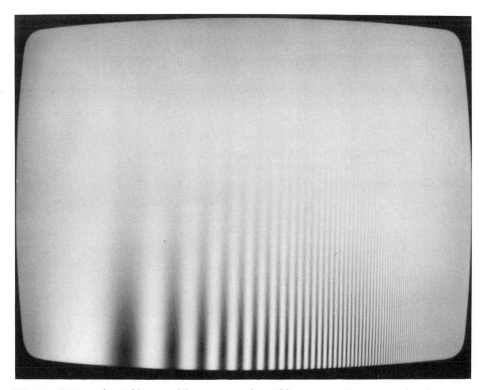

FIG. 3.4. Grating of variable spatial frequency, and variable contrast. One can see that the stripes are most visible in the middle, less visible on the left edge, and invisible on the right edge. Photograph provided by John Robson.

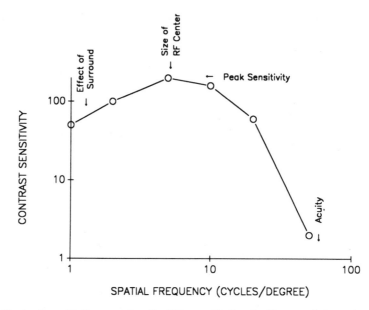

FIG. 3.5. Contrast sensitivity curve (see the "Glossary"). For significance of the various points on the curve, see the text.

The place where the curve meets the horizontal axis represents the finest grating that can be seen in any circumstances. This value of spatial frequency therefore corresponds to grating acuity. The peak of the curve shows the lowest contrast that can be detected at any spatial frequency. The fact that the curve drops at low spatial frequencies can be attributed to inhibitory lateral influences within the nervous system, because a stripe that is wide enough to activate lateral inhibition will produce a reduced response. Consequently, the position of the peak of the curve on the horizontal axis gives a reading of how wide a stripe has to be to sum excitatory influences without activating significant lateral inhibition as well.

All parts of the contrast sensitivity curve change with age (Atkinson et al., 1977; see Fig. 3.6). The high-frequency cutoff changes as predicted from acuity measurements. The contrast that can be detected decreases as the infant gets older, for all spatial frequencies. The low-frequency falloff becomes more pronounced with age. Also, the position of the peak of the curve shifts to higher spatial frequency with age. Use of the VEP, combined with a "sweep" stimulus that reduces the time required to accumulate data, gives higher sensitivity in young subjects, but the tendencies are the same (Norcia et al., 1990).

Many of these changes can be predicted, as can acuity changes, by the development of the cones in the fovea (Banks and Bennett, 1988; Wilson, 1988). The cones become longer with age, as well as narrower (Yuodelis and Hendrickson, 1986). In addition, the efficiency with which the inner segment funnels light into the outer segment increases. Both of these morphological alterations increase the efficiency of the cones for catching light, and consequently increase the contrast sensitivity.

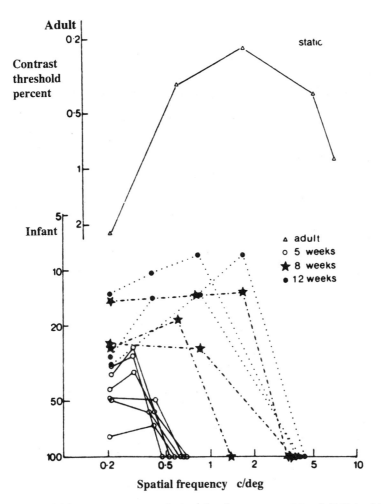

FIG. 3.6. Contrast sensitivity curves at 5, 8, and 12 weeks of age compared to adult. Data obtained from individual subjects by VEP technique. Reprinted with kind permission from Atkinson, J., Braddick, O., and Moar, K., 1977, Development of contrast sensitivity over the first 3 months of life in the human infant, *Vision Res.* **17**:1037–1044. Copyright 1977, Elsevier Science, Ltd., The Boulevard, Langford Lane, Kidlington OX5 1GB, UK.

There are three processes at work in the development of contrast sensitivity, each with a different time course: overall contrast sensitivity, contrast sensitivity at high spatial frequencies, and the low-frequency falloff. Between birth and 10 weeks of age, contrast sensitivity improves at all spatial frequencies (Norcia *et al.*, 1990). Further improvement after 10 weeks, lasting until 1 year of age or more, occurs primarily in contrast sensitivity to high spatial frequencies, leading to a further shift in the peak of the curve. The time course of the development of the low-frequency falloff is not so well established.

These three processes can be attributed to different mechanisms (Wilson, 1988). Overall sensitivity is related largely to the increase in the length of the photoreceptors, and the increase in funneling capacity. Increase in sensitivity at high spatial frequencies is related to packing of the foveal cones closer together as well as the increase in the percentage of the photons caught. The psychophysical results therefore suggest that the increase in the length of the cones should cease at around 10 weeks of age, and the increase in their packing density should continue after that. Unfortunately, the number of human retinas that have been studied is few, so that further work is needed to establish whether the time course of the development of the two relevant morphological properties matches the psychophysical properties appropriately. The lateral inhibitory mechanisms that explain the low-frequency falloff and their development will be discussed in Chapter 5.

C. Spatial Frequency Channels

The overall contrast sensitivity curve in the adult is made up of several channels sensitive to different spatial frequencies. These channels presumably correspond to cells that are tuned to different spatial frequencies. For example, cells in the P pathway respond to finer spatial frequencies than do cells in the M pathway. The existence of spatial frequency channels can be revealed by adaptation or masking experiments (e.g., Blakemore and Campbell, 1969). In a typical adaptation experiment, the subject looks at a particular spatial frequency for a period of time, and afterward the sensitivity for that spatial frequency and ones near it are reduced, while the sensitivity for higher and lower spatial frequencies are not. The experiment is similar to a color adaptation experiment, where there are cones tuned to different wavelengths, and stimulation of the red cones makes them less sensitive, so that the blue and green ones are relatively more sensitive. Spatial frequency adaptation experiments done in infants suggest that spatial frequency channels exist at an early age. This can be demonstrated at 6 weeks of age (Fiorentini *et al.*, 1983), with a larger effect at 12 weeks (Banks *et al.*, 1985). Whether all spatial frequency channels are there at birth, and whether some develop faster than others is not known, which is not surprising, because we do not know precisely how many spatial frequency channels there are in the adult.

D. Spectral Sensitivity and Wavelength Discrimination

Spectral sensitivity is affected by the growth in the length of the photoreceptors which, as we have discussed, results in an increase in the percentage of photons absorbed. For rod photoreceptors, this increase in length is approximately threefold (Drucker and Hendrickson, 1989). As a result, sensitivity in dim light is 1.7 log units below adult at 1 month of age, and 1 log unit below adult at 3 months of age, measured by the preferential-looking technique (Teller and Bornstein, 1987). Cone photoreceptors grow in length similarly, so that spectral sensitivity in the light-adapted state for the 2-month-old infant is also about ten times less than for the adult (Teller and Bornstein, 1987). The shape of the curve is approximately the same for infants and adults, but has a greater contribution at short wavelengths in some infants. This may be related to optical properties of the eye, rather than an increased contribution from the blue cones (Teller and Bornstein, 1987).

Infants can distinguish red from white at 2 months of age. They have both red-sensitive and green-sensitive cone pigments, as shown by Rayleigh matches, where a spectral yellow is matched to a mixture of spectral red and green (when both red and green pigments are present, a specific ratio of spectral red to spectral green is required; when only one pigment is present, a wide variety of ratios is acceptable). The blue cone pigment is also present: discriminations that use the blue cone pigment can be made, but are poor. Wavelength discrimination and saturation discrimination are poor compared to the adult (Teller and Bornstein, 1987), and this can also be explained by the smaller percentage of photons caught by the photoreceptors (Banks and Bennett, 1988). Thus, infants have red-, green-, and blue-absorbing cone pigments, and a normal pigment in the rods, just as in the adult, but their discriminative ability and sensitivity are poorer, because of the shorter length of the photoreceptors.

E. Dark Adaptation

It takes over half an hour for adults to get used to very dim light, and this is related to the long time required for the rod pigment to regenerate. This adaptation to the dark can be measured by changes in the diameter of the pupil, and by measuring the threshold for a criterion level of ERG. The time course in infants is the same as in the adult—about 400 sec (Hansen and Fulton, 1986; Fulton and Hansen, 1987)—so one concludes that the kinetics of the infant rod pigment are the same as in the adult.

F. Vernier Acuity

Vernier acuity is the ability to detect a misalignment of two lines. In the adult, vernier acuity is about 10 times better than grating acuity: that is, if the grating itself can be detected with lines spaced x min apart, the break will be detected with a displacement of x/10 min. Shimojo and Held (1987) investigated vernier acuity in 2- and 3-month-old infants, and found that whereas vernier acuity is better than grating acuity in the adult, it is worse than grating acuity in the infant before 11–12 weeks of age (for their stimulus, see Fig. 3.7). Thus, vernier acuity develops more rapidly than grating acuity with a crossover at this age (Fig. 3.8).

This rapid change may seem surprising, but there is an explanation. Vernier acuity increases faster than grating acuity with luminance, as predicted by Banks and Bennett (1988) from theoretical considerations. One would therefore expect infant vernier acuity to improve faster than grating acuity as the percentage of photons absorbed by the photoreceptors increases with age. In addition, vernier acuity is processed by modules of neurons that are located in the cortex. Vernier acuity falls off faster than grating acuity, as one moves the stimulus away from the fovea. Both retinal (Banks et al., 1991) and cortical (Levi et al., 1985) factors contribute to this. Poor sampling by cortical neurons in infants could therefore contribute to poor vernier acuity (Shimojo and Held, 1987).

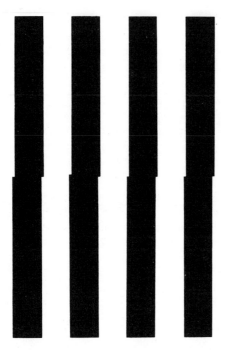

FIG. 3.7. Stimulus used by Shimojo and Held (1987) to test vernier acuity in infants.

Thus, there are two factors involved—improvement in the sensitivity of the photoreceptors and maturation of the visual cortex—and both contribute to the rapid increase of vernier acuity compared to grating acuity.

G. Orientation and Direction Sensitivity

Orientation discrimination depends very much on the stimulus and technique used. Newborns can discriminate the orientation of a stimulus if they are habituated to one orientation, then presented with a choice of two orientations side by side (Slater *et al.*, 1988). The discrimination is not made if the test orientations are presented sequentially. Results with a dynamic stimulus and the VEP show some development after birth (Braddick *et al.*, 1986). The dynamic stimulus consisted of a grating jittering 25 times per second in one orientation, followed by the same jitter with the perpendicular orientation. Three reversals of orientation per second give a noticeable response at 3 weeks of age, and eight reversals at 6 weeks of age. Clearly the infant has the cortical apparatus to detect orientations at birth, but this needs to mature before it can be seen in a gross response such as the VEP.

The VEP response to orientation is reduced if a second masking grating of slightly different spatial frequency is superimposed on the test grating. The effect in the adult depends on whether the masking grating is parallel or perpendicular to the test grating. When parallel, the response/contrast curve is shifted sideways; when perpendicular, the slope of the response/contrast curve is reduced. These two effects appear in infants at different times. The masking effect of the parallel grating is clear at 4 months of age, while the masking effect of the perpendicular grating is not clear until 10 months of age (Morrone and

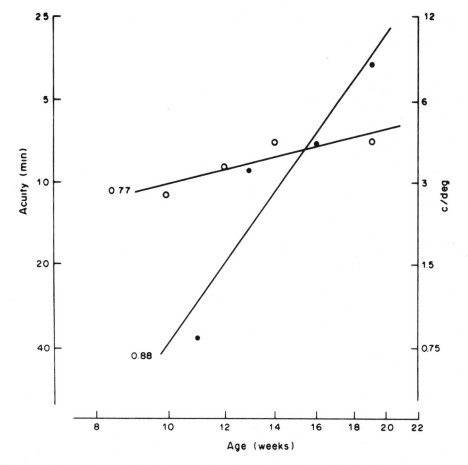

FIG. 3.8. Vernier acuity develops more rapidly than grating acuity in infants. Vernier acuity expressed in minutes of displacement (solid circles and left axis). Grating acuity expressed in cycles per degree (open circles and right axis). Reprinted with kind permission from Shimojo, S., and Held, R., 1987, Vernier acuity is less than grating acuity in 2- and 3.month-olds, *Vision Res.* **27**:77–86. Copyright 1987, Elsevier Science, Ltd., The Boulevard, Langford Lane, Kidlington OX5 1GB, UK.

Burr, 1986; see Fig. 3.9). There must be two different sets of connections in the cortex underlying these two effects, with different times of development.

Direction-specific responses must also be present at birth, because the newborn exhibits OKN. In order to detect the direction of movement to generate OKN, direction-specific cells are needed. However, like orientation-specific responses, they do not show up in the VEP until later on. A stimulus moving at 5°/sec is first noticeable at 10 weeks of age, and a stimulus moving at 20°/sec is first noticeable at 13 weeks (Wattam-Bell, 1991). The FPL technique, like the VEP, also does not demonstrate directional responses until some time after birth. As with orientation-specific responses, the apparatus must be there at birth, but matures with age and does not show up until later by the methods used.

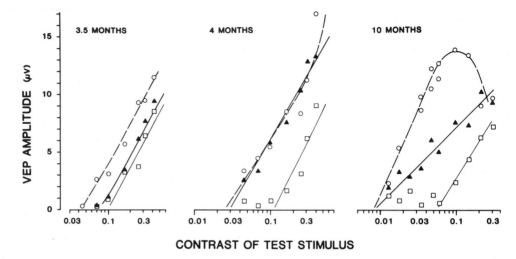

FIG. 3.9. Development of orientation masking. Curves plot the amplitude of the VEP response as a function of the contrast of the test stimulus, which was a grating of 1 cycle/degree. In the control state, there was no masking grating (○); with a parallel mask the curve was shifted sideways (□); and with a perpendicular mask the slope of the curve was reduced (▲). The masking effect of the parallel mask was noticeable at 4 months, and the masking effect of the perpendicular mask at 10 months. Reprinted with permission from Morrone, M. C., and Burr, D. C., 1986, Evidence for the existence and development of visual inhibition in humans, *Nature* **321**:235–237. Copyright 1986, MacMillan Magazines Limited.

H. Summary

Some visual properties are present at birth. Rhodopsin in the rod photo-receptors has a spectral sensitivity curve with the same shape as the adult, and regenerates with the same time course. All three cone pigments are present, and the light-adapted spectral sensitivity curve is close to that of the adult.

However, there are a number of properties that develop after birth. Several of these can be traced to the development of the cone photoreceptors in the fovea, which get longer and more tightly packed as the infant ages, and to the development of the rod photoreceptors around the fovea, which also get longer with age. These morphological changes play a large part between birth and a year of age in the improvement of acuity, contrast sensitivity, vernier acuity, and wavelength and saturation discrimination.

Other properties are present at birth, but mature in a quantitative way as the retina and cortex develop. This includes specificity for orientation and direction of movement, and perhaps also specificity of channels for different spatial frequencies. How this relates to the properties of the neurons in the central visual system will be discussed in Chapter 5.

III. Development of Binocular Vision

Getting the two eyes to work together is a complicated process. They must be able to converge or diverge, so that the two images of an object fall on corresponding parts of the two retinas. For this to occur accurately requires good acuity in both eyes, good control of eye movements, and the ability to tell whether an object is closer or farther away than the point of fixation. There must be good vision in both eyes, good connections between sensory and motor systems, and some depth perception.

Thus, there is a definite dependence of the various components of the system on each other during development. Vergence movements initially depend on cues other than stereopsis. Binocular function matures as the acuity in the retina matures and the vergence movements become more accurate. Development of the fine cue to depth perception, stereopsis, awaits the development of some binocular coordination. Stereopsis then enables yet more accurate vergence movements. When one thinks about it, logic virtually dictates that this must be the sequence of events.

A. Depth Perception

Helmholtz listed several cues to depth perception, some monocular, such as perspective, size, superposition, motion parallax, accommodation, and haze, and some binocular, such as stereopsis and convergence (see Glossary). To these can be added the gradients of texture studied by Gibson and his colleagues (1950), where coarse textures are seen as being closer than fine ones.

Unfortunately, it is extremely hard to study depth perception in very young infants. One of the first experiments on depth perception in infants was the "visual cliff," studied by Walk and Gibson (1961). Here the infant is placed at the center of a glass table so arranged that half of the table has a pattern immediately beneath the glass and appears solid, and half is transparent, allowing a view of the same pattern on the floor, suggesting a precipitous drop (Fig. 3.10). The observer studies whether the infant avoids the "cliff" when it moves away from the center. Because the test requires crawling, it cannot be done until several months of age, although some results can be obtained based on heart rate. At that stage, many but not all infants make the discrimination.

Yonas and his colleagues studied the response of infants to a number of different cues to depth perception (Yonas and Granrud, 1985). Much of their work was based on reaching by the infant with its hand to touch the object, which does not start until about 5 months of age. Their generalization was that infants respond to kinetic cues at 1–3 months of age, binocular cues at 3–5 months of age, and pictorial cues at 5–7 months of age. However, the only kinetic cue that they studied before the infant started to reach was an object expanding explosively, as though it would hit the infant. This elicited a blink reflex and head retraction. By binocular cues they meant stereopsis and convergence, which will be discussed below. Pictorial cues included size, texture gradient, shading, and interposition. It was clear that 7-month-old infants could respond to these as individual cues to depth perception.

There may be truth to the Yonas generalization. However, one wonders if infants might detect depth from some cues at an earlier age than they can physically respond to it with reaching responses. The crucial question from the developmental point of view is: what cues drive vergence movements early in life, to give good binocular coordination? Is this simply avoidance of diplopia,

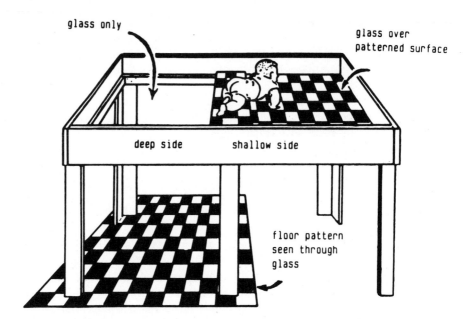

glass only

glass over
patterned surface

deep side   shallow side

floor pattern
seen through
glass

FIG. 3.10. The visual cliff. Infant is placed on divider and coaxed to go to a parent on either the "deep" or "shallow" side. Fewer descents to the deep side is taken as an indicator of depth perception. Reprinted with permission from Walk and Gibson (1961).

by some maximization of the response in binocular neurons? Or are cues to depth perception other than stereopsis involved? This remains to be tested thoroughly.

B. Orthotropia

Orthotropia is the ability of the two eyes to look together at an object, to give single vision. It can be measured by the Hirschberg test, in which reflections from the cornea are noted, in relation to the position of the pupil. For the results to be evaluated, one has to know the displacement of the corneal reflection from the optic axis or pupillary center (angle kappa), as well as the angle between the optic axis and the visual axis, which goes through the fovea.

One might assume that this is a straightforward procedure. In fact, the results have been rather difficult to obtain, and vary with different authors. However, the angle kappa varies with age, and when this is taken into account, the overall conclusion is that most infants are orthotropic, with some having the eyes turned outward a little, which is called exotropia (Thorn et al., 1994).

If infants were severely exotropic or esotropic (eye turned inward), they would have double vision (diplopia). This would obviously be a severe handicap. However, there are two factors that make diplopia less likely in an infant. The adult does not get diplopia unless the images in the eyes are separated by a certain amount—15 minutes of arc along the horizontal axis near the fixation point. The area giving single vision is called Panum's fusional area. Panum's fusional area has not been measured in the young infant, but from everything that we have discussed about the development of acuity and the eyeball, one would expect it to be larger than in the adult. The second factor relates to the development of the fovea. The fovea is not well developed at birth, and nobody really knows whether infants fixate with the center of their rod-free area, or some point nearby. In any case, from observations of the morphology, one would not expect the area of finest vision to be clearly positioned until the fovea develops, and the cones in the fovea have become densely packed. Consequently, a small degree of esotropia or exotropia can be tolerated in the infant, whereas it would not be in the adult.

C. Stereopsis

The most precise cue to depth perception depends on disparity and is called *stereopsis*. Disparity occurs when the two images fall on noncorresponding parts of the two retinas. For objects closer than the fixation point, the disparity is called *crossed* because the lines of sight cross each other between the eyes and the surface on which the eyes are focused. Conversely, the disparity is called *uncrossed* for objects farther away than the fixation point. As discussed in Chapter 2, there are cells in the adult visual cortex that respond to crossed disparity (near cells), and cells that respond to uncrossed disparity (far cells). Stereoscopic acuity in the adult, like vernier acuity, is better than grating acuity by a factor of approximately 10: one can detect a disparity of a few seconds of arc, whereas lines in a grating must be 1 or 2 minutes of arc apart before they are seen. One would therefore expect that some fineness of tuning in the retina, in the form of a certain level of grating acuity, would be required before such fine tuning in the cortex can occur.

The development of stereopsis has been given a great deal of attention, for several reasons. It can be assayed by a variety of techniques. There is a quantity, stereoscopic acuity, that can be measured. Moreover, it represents the onset of fine tuning in binocular function, and this onset is correlated with a number of other events.

Stereopsis can be measured using FPL and a pair of line displays. One display is arranged so that, for an adult, some lines appear to stand out in front of the others (Fig. 3.11). The other display is flat. The display with apparent depth becomes more interesting to the infant very suddenly around 16 weeks of age (Held *et al.*, 1980). When the infant makes the discrimination, stereoscopic acuity can be measured, and it increases from more than 60 minutes of arc to less than 1 minute of arc in a few weeks (Birch *et al.*, 1982; see Fig. 3.12A). Interestingly, the detection of crossed disparity develops earlier than that of uncrossed disparity (Fig. 3.12B).

Stereopsis can also be measured with random-dot stereograms. In these, there is a pattern of dots around the edge of the display that are identical for left and right eyes, and a pattern of dots in the center that are the same, but with a crossed or uncrossed displacement. For an adult, the center appears to stand out in front of or behind the plane of the edge pattern. A computer can be used to change the individual dots in a random way (dynamic stereogram), while keeping the left/right eye correlation, or to move the central display around to make it appear to move. FPL measurement of stereopsis, using a moving random-dot stereogram, also shows that stereopsis emerges at $3\frac{1}{2}$ to 6 months of

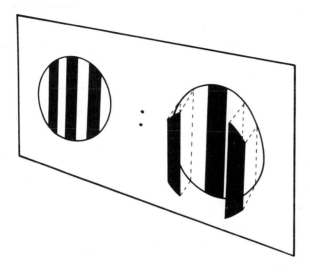

FIG. 3.11. Stimulus pair used to test stereopsis in infants. Two light-emitting diodes are in the center, with a flat display on the left, and a display with crossed disparity on the right (the dashed lines demonstrate the effect). Reprinted with permission from Held *et al.* (1980).

age (Fox *et al.*, 1980). A similar time course is found with both stationary and dynamic random-dot stereograms using the VEP (Braddick *et al.*, 1980; Petrig *et al.*, 1981).

Why does stereopsis appear so suddenly? Although the acuity and vergence movements that are needed to produce orthotropia obviously must reach a certain level of maturity before stereopsis can occur, improvement in grating acuity is small over the period during which stereopsis develops (compare Fig. 3.2 and 3.12), and there is an ability to converge before this time. Moreover, nothing in the development of the retina or the eye movement system would predict a different time of onset for crossed and uncrossed stereopsis. Schor (1985) argues that certain factors in monocular vision need to devel-

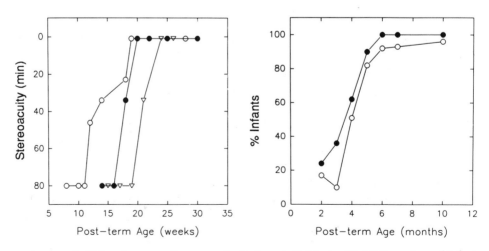

FIG. 3.12. (Left) Development of stereoacuity in three individuals. (Right) Percentage of infants who reached criterion for stereopsis when tested with crossed (●) or uncrossed (○) disparity. Data from Birch *et al.*, 1982.

op before stereopsis: small disparities are processed in the adult in spatial frequency channels tuned above 2.5 cycles/degree, and larger disparities are processed by lower spatial frequency channels. These channels may not be tuned adequately until 3 months of age. However, Schor's arguments aside, the most distinct correlation between the onset of stereopsis and another factor is with the segregation of ocular dominance columns.

D. The Correlation of the Onset of Stereopsis and Segregation of Ocular Dominance Columns

This correlation was first pointed out by Held and his colleagues (for review, see Held, 1993). The correlation has not been pinned down very well in the human, so we will have to anticipate Chapters 4 and 5, and present some evidence from the macaque monkey and the cat.

The segregation of ocular dominance columns occurs at the input layer of the visual cortex, which is layer IV. At birth, the afferents from the left and right eyes overlap, and synapse onto the same neurons in layer IV. Then, at a time that varies with the species, they segregate into separate left and right eye columns within layer IV, synapsing onto separate neurons. The convergence of the signals from the two eyes then occurs at the next level, which may be layers II and III, or layers V and VI. Thus, there is binocular convergence within primary visual cortex in both neonate and adult, but the layer and level at which it occurs is different.

Stereopsis in cats has been studied with a variation of the FPL technique, and an apparatus similar to the visual cliff (Timney, 1981). The kitten looks down on a pair of displays on the far side of a Plexiglas surface, and is made to jump down onto one side or the other (Fig. 3.13). There are monocular cues as

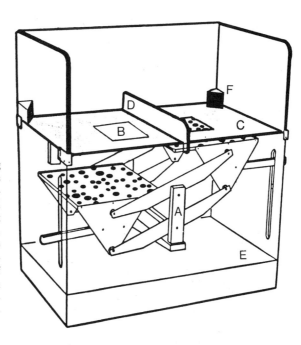

FIG. 3.13. Jumping stand for testing vision in kittens. There is a Plexiglas surface (B) with two masks on it. Below it, a display of dots can be moved to vary the relative distance of the left and right sides from the Plexiglas (A). A divider (D) forces the kitten to jump to one side or the other. Small speakers provide an audible indication of an incorrect choice. Reprinted with permission from *Investigative Ophthalmology and Visual Science*, Timney (1981).

well as binocular cues in this display, but most monocular cues are hidden by a mask. The disparity that can be detected with binocular viewing falls rapidly between 5 and 6 weeks of age as a result of stereoscopic mechanisms (Fig. 3.14). This is the same period of time over which the afferents from left and right eyes to the cortex are segregating (LeVay *et al.*, 1978).

Stereopsis in the macaque monkey has been studied with FPL and random-dot stereograms (O'Dell *et al.*, 1991). Stereopsis appears at a mean age of 4 weeks, and improves between then and 8 weeks of age. Again, this is the period of time over which the left and right eye afferents are segregating (LeVay *et al.*, 1980).

Unfortunately, the time at which geniculocortical afferents segregate in the human is not well established. However, in a preliminary report, Hickey found well-formed columns in a 6-month-old human infant, and poorly formed columns in a 4-month-old infant (Hickey and Peduzzi, 1987). Thus, there is a 2-month window during which segregation of afferents probably occurs. Since the experiments described above show that stereopsis emerges between 3 and 6 months, there is a reasonable correlation between development of stereopsis and segregation of ocular dominance columns in humans as well.

There are theoretical reasons to think that some binocular coordination of signals is required before cells sensitive to disparity develop. Sejnowski and his

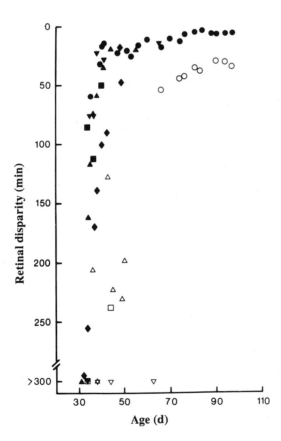

FIG. 3.14. Depth thresholds plotted as a function of age. Closed symbols, binocular thresholds; open symbols, monocular thresholds. Reprinted with permission from *Investigative Ophthalmology and Visual Science*, Timney (1981).

colleagues have modeled the conditions required (Berns et al., 1993). Their model shows that if there is correlation of activity within each eye but not between eyes, only monocular cells develop. If there is a small amount of correlation between the two eyes, only binocular zero disparity cells develop. If there is a two-phase model, starting with a period of correlations within each eye, followed by a period that includes correlations between the eyes, the model produces binocular cells sensitive for zero disparity and apparently monocular cells selective for nonzero disparity. The model thus supports the notion that a two-phase process is required for the development of stereopsis.

When a correlation like this between development of stereopsis and ocular dominance segregation has been found in three separate species, it indicates a significant general developmental process. This observation has led Held and his colleagues to look for other properties that might vary between the pre- and poststereoptic periods (Held, 1993).

E. The Pre- and Poststereoptic Periods

Two aspects of binocular summation differ between the pre- and post-stereoptic periods. Signals from the left and right eyes sum in their effect on the pupil in the adult. This can be seen by covering the left eye, observing the size of the pupil in the right eye, and observing whether the pupil contracts when the left eye is opened. Signals from the left eye start to have an effect on the size of the pupil in the right eye at 3 months of age, and the effect increases until adult summation is reached at 6 months of age (Birch and Held, 1983; see Fig. 3.15).

Signals from the left and right eyes also sum in the adult in their effect on acuity. Acuity is better by a factor of approximately $\sqrt{2}$ when both eyes are illuminated. This form of binocular summation also occurs in the poststereoptic period, but not in the prestereoptic period (Birch and Swanson, 1992).

Although these two forms of binocular summation correlate with the onset of stereopsis, the mechanism is unclear. According to signal/noise theory, de-

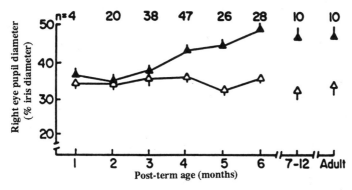

FIG. 3.15. Difference in pupil diameter in right eye with left eye occluded (▲), and with left eye open (△). The number of infants tested at each age is indicated along the top of the figure. Reprinted with permission from *Investigative Ophthalmology and Visual Science*, Birch and Held (1983).

tectability improves with summation of two signals if they have separate sources of noise, but not if they have a common form of noise. Birch and her colleagues have used this point as an explanation for their findings. However, most "noise" in the visual system comes from the retina, and there are separate sources of noise from the left and right eyes both before and after stereopsis occurs. What changes is the level at which the signals and their noise are combined, not the nature of the noise. Whatever the explanation, the correlation of binocular summation with stereopsis is most intriguing.

Another property that emerges with stereopsis is the avoidance of "rivalrous stimuli." Rivalrous stimuli are stimuli that differ in form or color in the two eyes, cannot be fused into a single perception, and are seen as an alternation between the left and right eye images. Infants will avoid checkerboards and random-dot patterns that appear rivalrous to an adult, but not until they reach the poststereoptic period (Birch *et al.*, 1985). Even more intriguingly, infants may *prefer* a stimulus that is rivalrous to an adult in the prestereoptic period. For example, consider vertical lines presented to the left eye and horizontal lines presented to the right eye, as shown to an infant on the left screen (Fig. 3.16). This can be fused into a single stimulus (binocular 2) or seen as rivalrous (binocular 1). Vertical lines presented to both eyes (right screen, Fig. 3.16) will clearly be fused as vertical lines in all cases. Using FPL, infants prefer the left screen in the prestereoptic period, presumably because they see the fused

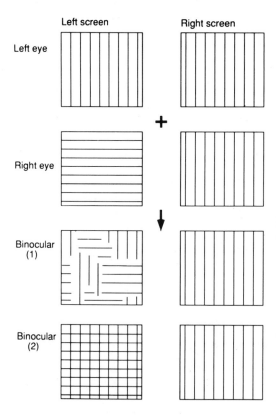

FIG. 3.16. Stimulus to test fusion versus rivalry. Top two displays show the stimuli. The third display (binocular 1) shows what is expected when rivalry is seen in the left screen; the fourth display (binocular 2) shows what is expected when the two images on the left screen are fused. Reprinted with kind permission from Shimojo, S., Bauer, J., O'Connell, K. M., and Held, R., 1986, Prestereoptic binocular vision in infants, *Vision Res.* **26**:501–510. Copyright 1986, Elsevier Science, Ltd., The Boulevard, Langford Lane, Kidlington OX5 1GB, UK.

percept (binocular 2) and regard it as more interesting (Shimojo et al., 1986). In the poststereoptic period, they prefer the right screen, presumably because the left screen has become rivalrous and is unpleasant.

Obviously the full explanation for these results depends on what is analyzed by the cells in layer IV. Properties first calculated in layer IV may be fused in the prestereoptic period, when the calculation is made after the signals from the eyes converge, and appear rivalrous in the poststereoptic period, when the calculation is made before the left and right eye signals are combined. Thus, we speculate that when left and right eyes converge in layer IV, and orientation is analyzed at the same time, a checkerboard is seen (binocular 2), but when orientation is analyzed in layer IV before signals from the left and right eyes converge, rivalry will occur.

More important than either summation or rivalry for the function of the visual system are vergence movements and orthotropia. Although both vergence movements and orthotropia are present before stereopsis, orthotropia shows some improvement, and vergence movements show considerable quantitative improvement, with the onset of stereopsis. Full convergence, as judged by the ability of the infant to follow a toy to within 12 cm of its face, appears between 8 and 16 weeks of age (Thorn et al., 1994). Orthotropia, as judged by some observers, is not complete until 12 weeks of age. Measurements of both orthotropia and vergence movements are subject to experimental inaccuracies, which are larger than the stereoscopic signals that can drive them when stereoscopic acuity reaches 1 minute of arc. Consequently, it seems likely that the accuracy with which an infant can focus on an object improves beyond the limits of experimental error when stereoscopic acuity reaches its finest level of tuning.

F. Summary

These results show that the order in which events occur in the development of binocular vision is a logical one. At birth, the fovea is immature, and grating acuity is poor, but the eyes look in approximately the same direction. The neonatal infant presumably does not have diplopia, but the eyes do not have to be as precisely aligned as they do in the adult to avoid this. Soon after birth, there is some binocular coordination, and there is consequently some ability to make vergence movements.

Over the first 3 months the fovea matures, grating acuity improves, and the eyes become more able to fixate together on an object. Presumably, cells in layer IV of the cortex are acquiring characteristics that will enable them to act as an appropriate input to near and far cells after stereopsis occurs.

Then, between 3 and 6 months of age, dramatic alterations occur in the visual cortex, and in the ability of the eyes to work together. Stereopsis becomes detectable, followed by a rapid increase in stereoscopic acuity. The eyes develop the ability to make full convergence movements. Orthotropia is mature. Binocular summation occurs, and some stimuli that were previously fused become rivalrous.

After 6 months of age there is further development in some visual properties. Grating acuity, for example, continues to improve. However, the main aspects of binocular development are complete when stereoscopic acuity and all of the functions that it governs reaches 1 minute of arc.

IV. Development of Eye Movements

Some aspects of the development of eye movements have already been discussed, primarily those aspects that relate to the development of binocular function, such as vergence movements and the ability to fixate on an object. Nevertheless, it is useful to give some details. Other aspects, such as smooth pursuit movements and saccadic movements, remain to be discussed.

A. Fixation and Refixation

The duration of fixation in infants is short for images rich in detail. This might be expected, as the infant is interested in exploring, and an image rich in detail contains more to explore. The drift away from fixation is greater in images with detail, and so is the tendency to make a new fixation (Hainline, 1993). These processes become more sophisticated as recognition and memory develop (Bronson, 1982).

Refixation varies from infant to infant, and so it does in uninstructed adults also (Hainline *et al.*, 1990). Figure 3.17 shows results from three infants and

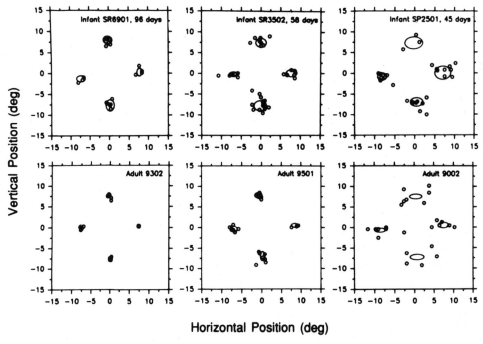

FIG. 3.17. Refixation movements in three infants and three adults. Subjects made saccades to objects 7.5° away from the center above, below, left, or right of the center. From Hainline *et al.* (1990, Fig. 3).

three adults, when the subjects shifted their gaze to one of four targets 7.5° from the initial fixation point. The one infant who showed a performance comparable to the better adults was 14 weeks of age, and probably into the stereoptic period.

B. Saccades

Saccadic eye movements in infants can be almost as fast as in adults (400°/sec), if the stimuli grab the infant's attention (Hainline et al., 1984). Saccades when looking at textures that fill the whole screen can be quite mature (Fig. 3.18). Saccades to forms such as squares, circles, and triangles are less mature. For less interesting stimuli, the infant may make a series of saccades, rather than a single large one (Aslin and Salapatek, 1975; Roucoux et al., 1983).

Two differences between saccades in infants and saccades in adults are noticeable (Hainline, 1993). Saccades in infants sometimes occur with less than 200 msec between them (see Fig. 3.18, infant LV). This almost never occurs in the adult. The infant also sometimes shows an oscillatory eye movement, where the eyes saccade away from an object and then back again (see Fig. 3.18, infant BK). This is only seen in adults in pathological conditions.

C. Smooth Pursuit

Smooth pursuit eye movements are essentially fixation on a moving target. Indeed, adults cannot make smooth pursuit eye movements, unless there is a

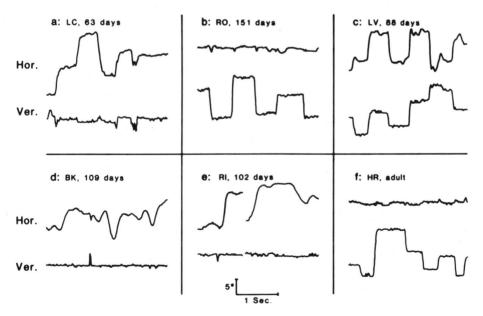

FIG. 3.18. Saccadic eye movements in five infants and one adult. Reprinted with kind permission from Hainline, L., Turkel, J., Abramov, L., Lemerise, E., and Harris, C. M., 1984, Characteristics of saccades in human infants, *Vision Res.* **24:**1771–1780. Copyright 1984, Elsevier Science, Ltd., The Boulevard, Langford Lane, Kidlington OX5 1GB, UK.

target to follow. Smooth pursuit therefore requires the ability to fixate, and the ability to detect movement.

Infants show smooth pursuit movements to slowly moving targets. The maximum velocity that can be followed increases with age (Roucoux *et al.*, 1983). When this velocity is exceeded, the infant may still be able to keep up, but will use a mixture of smooth pursuit and saccades (Hainline, 1993). The results depend on the target—whether it is a large one, such as a face, or unpatterned spots, circles, or bars.

D. Vergence

As discussed above, some vergence movements are seen at 1 month of age, and more pronounced movements at 2 and 3 months (Aslin, 1977). These occur in response to an object moved slowly toward or away from the infant. A large improvement in the number of adequate vergence movements occurs at 4–5 months of age (Mitkin and Orestova, 1988).

Another stimulus that is used to elicit a vergence movement in the adult is placing a base-out prism in front of one eye. The prism causes a vergence movement to keep the two eyes fixated together on the object that the adult is looking at. However, such a prism will not elicit a vergence movement in the infant. It could be that the infant notices the edge of the prism and is distracted by that, since he/she has not been instructed to keep their gaze fixed on some object in the distance. However, the test pits the stereoscopic cue for depth perception against any monocular cues that may be present. Consequently, before the onset of stereopsis, the infant would not be expected to respond to this test.

E. Optokinetic Nystagmus

OKN is elicited by a large stimulus covering a substantial amount of the visual field, and can be found in the newborn. The eyes follow the stimulus for a period of time, then flick back in a fast saccadic-like movement. Infants can follow the stimulus better for a stimulus moving in the nasal direction than for one moving in the temporal direction (Naegele and Held, 1982). Interestingly, this direction-dependent asymmetry disappears at around 5 months of age. OKN is at least partly a subcortical phenomenon. Perhaps, after stereopsis is established at 5 months, the cortex exerts some control to make the gain of the responses in the two directions equal. However, alternative explanations cannot be ruled out.

F. Summary

Several eye movement properties develop in synchrony with the sensory parts of the visual system. The ability to fixate improves as the fovea and acuity develop. The ability to make smooth pursuit eye movements, as opposed to saccades that keep the eyes up with the stimulus, improves as the ability to detect the velocity of a moving stimulus improves. Vergence movements improve as depth perception becomes more acute.

On the other hand, saccadic eye movements show changes that are not related to sensory properties. These are establishment of a 200-msec delay between saccades, disappearance of oscillatory movements away from the object and back again, and establishment of a single large saccade to small targets far away, as opposed to several smaller saccades. The crucial component in the development of these properties is most likely in the brain stem, rather than in the afferent pathways.

V. Pattern Perception

There is a considerable literature on pattern perception in infants, which has been reviewed in several volumes (see Banks and Salapatek, 1983; Salapatek and Cohen, 1987; Weiss and Zelazo, 1991). It will not be reviewed in this book, because my prime purpose is to correlate behavioral and psychophysical properties with anatomy and physiology during development, and to show how these properties are disrupted by the effects of visual deprivation. Unfortunately, our understanding of the anatomy and physiology of the visual system has not yet reached the point where more complicated aspects of pattern perception are understood in a detailed way. Hopefully another book like this one will be able to address pattern perception, as well as the psychophysical properties dealt with above, in 10 to 20 year's time.

References

Aslin, R. N., 1977, Development of binocular fixation in human infants, *J. Exp. Child Psychol.* **23**:133–150.

Aslin, R. N., and Salapatek, P., 1975, Saccadic localization of visual targets by the very young human infant, *Percept. Psychophys.* **17**:293–302.

Atkinson, J., Braddick, O., and Moar, K., 1977, Development of contrast sensitivity over the first 3 months of life in the human infant, *Vision Res.* **17**:1037–1044.

Banks, M. S., 1980, The development of visual accommodation during early infancy, *Child Dev.* **51**:646–666.

Banks, M. S., and Bennett, P. J., 1988, Optical and photoreceptor immaturities limit the spatial and chromatic vision of human neonates, *J. Opt. Soc. Am. [A]* **5**:2059–2079.

Banks, M. S., and Salapatek, P., 1983, Infant visual perception, in: *Handbook of Child Psychology II. Infancy and Developmental Psychobiology* (P. H. Mussen, ed.), Wiley, New York, pp. 435–571.

Banks, M. S., Stephens, P. R., and Hartmann, E. E., 1985, The development of basic mechanisms of pattern vision: Spatial frequency channels, *J. Exp. Child Psychol.* **40**:501–527.

Banks, M. S., Sekuler, A. B., and Anderson, S. J., 1991, Peripheral spatial vision: Limits imposed by optics, photoreceptors, and receptor pooling, *J. Opt. Soc. Am. [A]* **8**:1775–1787.

Berns, G. S., Dayan, P., and Sejnowski, T. J., 1993, A correlational model for the development of disparity selectivity in visual cortex that depends on prenatal and postnatal phases, *Proc. Natl. Acad. Sci. USA* **90**:8277–8281.

Birch, E. E., 1993, Stereopsis in infants and its developmental relation to visual acuity, in: *Early Visual Development, Normal and Abnormal* (K. Simons, ed.), Oxford University Press, London, pp. 224–236.

Birch, E. E., and Held, R., 1983, The development of binocular summation in human infants, *Invest. Ophthalmol. Vis. Sci.* **24**:1103–1107.

Birch, E. E., and Swanson, W. H., 1992, Probability summation of acuity in the human infant, *Vision Res.* **32**:1999–2003.

Birch, E. E., Gwiazda, J., and Held, R., 1982, Stereoacuity development for crossed and uncrossed disparities in human infants, *Vision Res.* **22**:507–513.

Birch, E. E., Shimojo, S., and Held, R., 1985, Preferential-looking assessment of fusion and stereopsis in infants aged 1–6 months, *Invest. Ophthalmol. Vis. Sci.* **26**:366–370.

Blakemore, C., and Campbell, F. W., 1969, On the existence of neurones in the human visual system selectively sensitive to the orientation and size of retinal images, *J. Physiol. (London)* **203**:237–260.

Braddick, O., Atkinson, J., Julesz, B., Kropfl, W., Bodis-Wollner, I., and Raab, E., 1980, Cortical binocularity in infants, *Nature* **288**:363–365.

Braddick, O., Wattam-Bell, J., and Atkinson, J., 1986, Orientation-specific cortical responses develop in early infancy, *Nature* **320**:617–619.

Bronson, G. W., 1982, *The Scanning Patterns of Human Infants: Implications for Visual Learning*, Ablex, Norwood, NJ.

Dobson, V., and Teller, D. Y., 1978, Visual acuity in human infants: A review and comparison of behavioral and electrophysiological studies, *Vision Res.* **18**:1469–1483.

Drucker, D. N., and Hendrickson, A. E., 1989, The morphological development of extrafoveal human retina, *Invest. Ophthalmol. Vis. Sci.* **30**:226.

Fiorentini, A., Pirchio, M., and Spinelli, D., 1983, Electrophysiological evidence for spatial frequency selective mechanisms in adults and infants, *Vision Res.* **23**:119–127.

Fox, R., Aslin, R. N., Shea, S. L., and Dumais, S. T., 1980, Stereopsis in human infants, *Science* **207**:323–324.

Fulton, A. B., and Hansen, R. M., 1987, The relationship of retinal sensitivity and rhodopsin in human infants, *Vision Res.* **27**:697–704.

Gibson, J. J., 1950, *The Perception of the Visual World*, Houghton Mifflin, Boston.

Hainline, L., 1993, Conjugate eye movements of infants, in: *Early Visual Development, Normal and Abnormal* (K. Simons, ed.), Oxford University Press, London, pp. 47–79.

Hainline, L., Turkel, J., Abramov, I., Lemerise, E., and Harris, C. M., 1984, Characteristics of saccades in human infants, *Vision Res.* **24**:1771–1780.

Hainline, L., Harris, C. M., and Krinsky, S., 1990, Variability of refixations in infants, *Infant Behav. Dev.* **13**:321–342.

Hansen, R. M., and Fulton, A. B., 1986, Pupillary changes during dark adaptation in human infants, *Invest. Ophthalmol. Vis. Sci.* **27**:1726–1729.

Held, R., 1993, Two stages in the development of binocular vision and eye alignment, in: *Early Visual Development, Normal and Abnormal* (K. Simons, ed.), Oxford University Press, London, pp. 250–257.

Held, R., Birch, E. E., and Gwiazda, J., 1980, Stereoacuity of human infants, *Proc. Natl. Acad. Sci. USA* **77**:5572–5574.

Hickey, T. L., and Peduzzi, J. D., 1987, Structure and development of the visual system, in: *Handbook of Infant Perception* (P. Salapatek and L. Cohen, eds.), Academic Press, New York, pp. 1–42.

Howland, H. C., 1993, Early refractive development, in: *Early Visual Development, Normal and Abnormal* (K. Simons, ed.), Oxford University Press, London, pp. 5–13.

Katz, B., and Sireteanu, R., 1990, The Teller acuity card test: A useful method for the clinical routine? *Clin. Vis. Sci.* **5**:307–323.

LeVay, S., Stryker, M. P., and Shatz, C. J., 1978, Ocular dominance columns and their development in layer IV of the cat's visual cortex: A quantitative study, *J. Comp. Neurol.* **179**:223–244.

LeVay, S., Wiesel, T. N., and Hubel, D. H., 1980, The development of ocular dominance columns in normal and visually deprived monkeys, *J. Comp. Neurol.* **191**:1–51.

Levi, D. M., Klein, S. A., and Aitsebaomo, A. P., 1985, Vernier acuity, crowding and cortical magnification, *Vision Res.* **25**:963–977.

Mitkin, A., and Orestova, E., 1988, Development of binocular vision in early ontogenesis, *Psychol. Beitr.* **30**:65–74.

Morrone, M. D., and Burr, D. C., 1986, Evidence for the existence and development of visual inhibition in humans, *Nature* **321**:235–237.

Naegele, J. R., and Held, R., 1982, The postnatal development of monocular optokinetic nystagmus in infants, *Vision Res.* **22**:341–346.

Norcia, A. M., and Tyler, C. W., 1985, Spatial frequency sweep VEP: Visual acuity during the first year of life, *Vision Res.* **25**:1399–1408.

Norcia, A. M., Tyler, C. W., and Hamer, R. D., 1990, Development of contrast sensitivity in the human infant, *Vision Res.* **30**:1475–1486.

O'Dell, C. D., Quick, M. W., and Boothe, R. G., 1991, The development of stereoacuity in infant rhesus monkeys, *Invest. Ophthalmol. Vis. Sci.* **32**:1044.

Petrig, B., Julesz, B., Kropfl, W., Baumgartner, G., and Anliker, M., 1981, Development of stereopsis and cortical binocularity in human infants: Electrophysiological evidence, *Science* **213**:1402–1405.

Roucoux, A., Culee, C., and Roucoux, M., 1983, Development of fixation and pursuit eye movements in human infants, *Behav. Brain Res.* **10**:133–139.

Salapatek, P., and Cohen, L., 1987, *Handbook of Infant Perception*, Academic Press, New York.

Schor, C. M., 1985, Development of stereopsis depends upon contrast sensitivity and spatial tuning, *J. Am. Optom. Assoc.* **56**:628–635.

Shimojo, S., 1993, Development of interocular vision in infants, in: *Early Visual Development, Normal and Abnormal* (K. Simons, ed.), Oxford University Press, London, pp. 201–223.

Shimojo, S., and Held, R., 1987, Vernier acuity is less than grating acuity in 2- and 3-month-olds, *Vision Res.* **27**:77–86.

Shimojo, S., Bauer, J., O'Connell, K. M., and Held, R., 1986, Pre-stereoptic binocular vision in infants, *Vision Res.* **26**:501–510.

Slater, A. M., Morison, V., and Somers, M., 1988, Orientation discrimination and cortical function in the human newborn, *Perception* **17**:597–602.

Teller, D. Y., 1977, The forced-choice preferential looking procedure: A psychophysical technique for use with human infants, *Infant Behav. Dev.* **2**:135–153.

Teller, D. Y., and Bornstein, M. H., 1987, Infant color vision and color perception, in: *Handbook of Infant Perception* (P. Salapatek and L. Cohen, eds.), Academic Press, New York.

Thorn, F., Gwiazda, J., Cruz, A., Bauer, J., and Held, R., 1994, The development of eye alignment, convergence, and sensory binocularity in young infants, *Invest. Ophthalmol. Vis. Sci.* **35**:544–553.

Timney, B. N., 1981, Development of binocular depth perception in kittens, *Invest. Ophthalmol. Vis. Sci.* **21**:493–496.

Walk, R. D., and Gibson, E. J., 1961, A comparative and analytical study of visual depth perception, *Psychol. Monogr.* **75**:1–44.

Wattam-Bell, J., 1991, Development of motion-specific cortical responses in infancy, *Vision Res.* **31**:287–297.

Weiss, M. J., and Zelazo, P. R., 1991, *Newborn Attention*, Ablex, Norwood, NJ.

Wilson, H. R., 1988, Development of spatiotemporal mechanisms in the human infant, *Vision Res.* **28**:611–628.

Yonas, A., and Granrud, C. E., 1985, The development of sensitivity to kinetic, binocular and pictorial depth information in human infants, in: *Brain Mechanisms and Spatial Vision* (D. Ingle, D. Lee, and R. M. Jeannerod, eds.), Nijhoff, The Hague.

Yuodelis, C., and Hendrickson, A., 1986, A qualitative and quantitative analysis of the human fovea during development, *Vision Res.* **26**:847–855.

4

Anatomical Development of the Visual System

The development of the nervous system is a complex and astounding phenomenon. The human nervous system consists of over ten billion cells, and each has its own individual job to do. Cells in the various parts of the nervous system are generated over the same period, and their projections grow out simultaneously but in different directions. Somehow these billions of projections have to cross a plethora of other fibers along the way, in many cases traversing a long distance, in order to find their way to the right nucleus and finally to the right cells in the nucleus.

An orderly sequence of steps is involved. The cells must first be generated, then migrate to their appropriate, often distant destination. They form dendrites to receive their inputs, and axons to transmit their outputs, sometimes while the cell bodies are still migrating. The axons find their way to the correct target structure, and form an orderly pattern within that nucleus. The brain produces more cells than are used in the mature organism, and there may be a loss of many cells that project to an inappropriate nucleus. Connections are made between a cell and its target, then the connections are refined by a process of pruning of dendrites, retraction of axonal terminals, sprouting of new terminals, and changing of synapses.

The initial steps are under chemical or molecular control, as suggested by Sperry in his celebrated chemoaffinity hypothesis that was based on many observations made by early embryologists (Sperry, 1963). Molecular cues guide fibers toward the appropriate target and keep them away from inappropriate ones by mechanisms of repulsion and attraction. This governs development before the synaptic connections are made, and before there is sensory input or motor output. Later steps are influenced by electrical activity between cells in the system. Activity governs the refinement of the strength and distribution of connections, to make them conform to the correct quantitative analysis of sensory signals and control of movement. Consequently, we can define two periods in the development of the nervous system: in the first, genetic factors provide the molecular instructions, and in the second, environmental factors control the refinement of connections. During the second period the system is said to be mutable or "plastic," and we talk about "experience-dependent plasticity" in the nervous system as a whole, and for the visual system, "sensory-dependent plasticity."

This whole process of development and plasticity has been most thoroughly studied in the visual system. We will concentrate on the mammalian visual system, because that is where correlations can best be made between the anatomy, the physiology, and the psychophysical properties described in Chapter 3, and the similarity to human vision is most obvious. Considerable work has also been done on the development of connections between the retina and tectum of amphibians. Some of that work will be discussed later, under the heading of the mechanisms involved in development.

Cells in the three main bodies of the sensory part of the mammalian visual system—the retina, lateral geniculate nucleus, and visual cortex—are generated during overlapping periods of embryonic development. For example, cells in the retina are generated in the macaque monkey between embryonic day 30 and embryonic day 120 (E30–E120), in the lateral geniculate nucleus between E36 and E43, and in the cortex between E40 and E90 (Rakic, 1992). The comparatively long period of cell generation in the retina occurs because there is a gradient of cell generation within the retina, the central part near the fovea being generated first and peripheral parts later (LaVail et al., 1991).

Cells destined for the visual cortex are generated in a pattern that has important consequences for the organization of the cortex. Cortical neurons are generated from stem cells located in a layer in the deepest part of the cortex called the ventricular zone. The young neurons migrate away from the ventricular zone to form the cortical layers (Fig. 4.1). The first cells to be generated are temporary, and eventually die. Some migrate to layer I, and some to the white matter below what will become layer VI (Marin-Padilla, 1971; Rakic, 1977; Luskin and Shatz, 1985; Kostovic and Rakic, 1990). Those in layer I are known as Cajal–Retzius cells, and those below layer VI as subplate cells. The cortex itself is generated after these transitory cells in an inside-out fashion. As illustrated in Fig. 4.1, the innermost layer, layer VI, is generated first, followed in sequential order by layer V, layer IV, layer III, and finally the outermost layer, which is layer II (Rakic, 1974; Luskin and Shatz, 1985). Since the cells are generated in the ventricular zone, below layer VI, the consequence is that cells migrate past the lower layers as they move to their final position. The whole process is a slow one. In the cat the process starts halfway through gestation at E30, and the cells for layer II do not reach their final position until 2 weeks after birth (Shatz and Luskin, 1986; see Fig. 4.2).

As the cells move through the layers, they are closely apposed to glial cells, called radial glia, which guide the young neurons away from the ventricular zone (Rakic, 1972; see Fig. 4.3). The young neurons develop into mature cells, the majority of whose axons and dendrites are lined up radially within the cortex. Indeed, observation of this organization by Lorente de Nó (1954) led him to propose that the cortex is arranged in a columnar fashion, long before the physiological evidence mentioned earlier came along. It seems likely that the radial migration of cells during development has something to do with the columnar organization of cortex, although the exact mechanism for this has not yet been worked out.

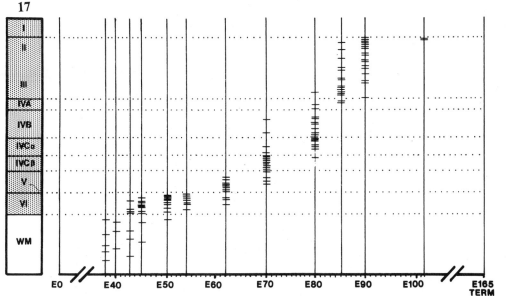

FIG. 4.1. Birthdates of neurons destined for various layers in the monkey visual cortex. The layers are numbered on the left. Each line represents a single neuron that was labeled with [³H]thymidine at the age shown, with its position determined at 2–5 months after birth. Neurons ending up in white matter (WM) are the remnant of the subplate neurons. Modified with permission from Rakic, P., 1974, Neurons in rhesus monkey visual cortex: Systematic relation between time of origin and eventual disposition, *Science* **183**:425–427. Copyright 1974, American Association for the Advancement of Science.

Some cells migrate tangentially (Walsh and Cepko, 1988). Whether this has any influence on the development of connections within the cortex is not clear. It can occur within the ventricular zone before radial migration starts. It can also occur after cells have left the ventricular zone, particularly in lateral parts of the cortex (Austin and Cepko, 1990). Lateral connections within the cortex tend to be short ones, with the exception of a few in layers II/III and VI that connect columns with similar properties. It would make sense for the cells that make long-distance lateral connections to be the ones that migrate tangentially after they have left the ventricular zone, but whether this is so is not yet known.

I. Organization under Genetic and Molecular Control

As a general rule, cells in the visual system project to approximately the correct location under genetic and molecular control. We do not know the identities of the genes or the molecules, but we do know that axons find the correct targets, the correct general area within the target, and sometimes the correct layer within the target. There are some genetic defects that can affect this routing. For example, albino animals and humans have an abnormality at the optic chiasm, such that too many fibers project to the contralateral lateral

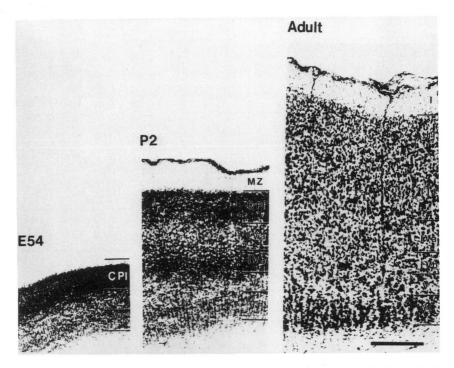

FIG. 4.2. Genesis of visual cortex in the cat. At E54, layers V and VI are formed; 2 days after birth, at P2, layer IV is formed but layers II and III are not. MZ, marginal zone; CPI, cortical plate. Reprinted with permission from Payne *et al.*, 1988, Development of connections in cat visual and auditory cortex, in: *Cerebral Cortex: Development and Maturation of Cerebral Cortex*, Plenum Press.

geniculate nucleus, and too few to the ipsilateral geniculate (Guillery, 1974). This results in an abnormality in coordination of the two halves of the field of view. Normally, the left side of the brain deals with the right half of the field of view, and the right side of the brain deals with the left half of the field of view. Because of the abnormal crossing in the chiasm, some fibers dealing with the left half of the field of view in albinos will reach the left side of the brain, and similarly for the right.

Long-distance connections between different areas dealing with vision are largely determined by molecular cues. Fibers from the retina project to the thalamus and terminate in the lateral geniculate nucleus, but not in the medial geniculate nucleus, although it is near their pathway. Fibers from the lateral geniculate nucleus project to area 17 in the macaque monkey, but very few to area 18, which is immediately adjacent (Rakic, 1977; see Fig. 4.4). Fibers from cells in layer VI of the cortex, which project back to the lateral geniculate nucleus, are generated while the layer VI cells are still differentiating, before the afferents to the cortex reach their target in layer IV (Shatz and Rakic, 1981). Thus, afferents to the cortex and efferents from the cortex pass each other in the white matter, and may help to guide each other.

Cells in the subplate below the cortex have a significant role in the path-finding of the afferent fibers. Axons from the lateral geniculate nucleus grow

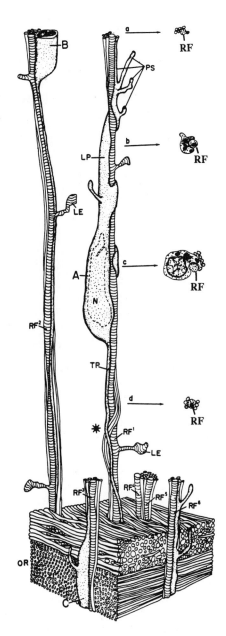

FIG. 4.3. Neurons (A, B, C) migrating through the cortex from the ventricular zone below toward the surface above, in close apposition to radial glia cells (RF). Neuron A is shown with its leading process (LP), pseudopodia (PS), and trailing process (TP). Cross sections at four levels are shown on the right. The neurons are in close contact with the radial glia at all levels. OR, optic radiation. Reprinted with permission from Rakic, P., 1972, Mode of cell migration to the superficial layers of fetal monkey neocortex, *J. Comp. Neurol.* **145**:61–83. Copyright 1972, John Wiley & Sons, Inc.

toward the cortex in the subplate (Rakic, 1976; Shatz and Luskin, 1986). When the axons reach the correct general location, they stop in the subplate for a period of time termed the "waiting period" by Rakic (1977). This wait may last several weeks in the slowly developing primate brain. At this stage, axons from the geniculate make connections with the subplate cells. The subplate cells have axons that contact cells in layer IV; consequently, the subplate cells can be stimulated monosynaptically from the lateral geniculate nucleus, while layer IV is stimulated polysynaptically (Friauf *et al.,* 1990). In the cat the connection

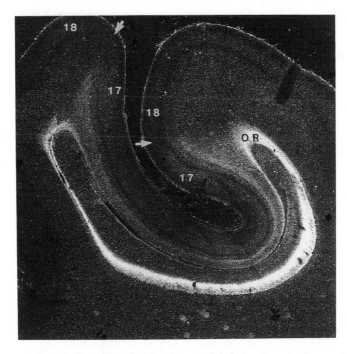

FIG. 4.4. Geniculocortical afferents to the visual cortex labeled at E110 in the monkey, and visualized at E124. The optic radiation (OR) sends axons only to area 17. Projections to the cortex stop sharply at the borderline between area 17 and area 18 (arrows). Some axons or terminals have invaded the cortical plate, but are distributed uniformly over layers IV and VI. Modified with permission from Rakic, P., 1976, Prenatal genesis of connections subserving ocular dominance in the rhesus monkey, *Nature* **261**:467–471. Copyright 1976, MacMillan Magazines Limited.

to layer IV is polysynaptic at birth, the geniculate fibers grow into layer IV after birth (Shatz and Luskin, 1986), and the connections to layer IV become monosynaptic at some time before postnatal day 21 (Friauf and Shatz, 1991; see Fig. 4.5). If the subplate cells are deleted, the lateral geniculate fibers go past their correct location, and end up somewhere else (Ghosh *et al.*, 1990; see Fig. 4.6). Thus, the subplate cells probably contain the molecular cues concerning the correct location for the afferent fibers. This may be their prime function, because many of them die soon after the lateral geniculate fibers make contact with them (Chun and Shatz, 1989; Kostovic and Rakic, 1990).

The organization of layers within visual cortex is also controlled by molecular cues. Afferents enter layer IV, efferents project back to the lateral geniculate from layer VI, and efferents to the superior colliculus come from layer V. This specificity is retained when slices of cortex and lateral geniculate or superior colliculus are placed in a culture dish (Yamamoto *et al.*, 1989; Blakemore and Molnar, 1990; Novak and Bolz, 1993; see Fig. 4.7). The slice of lateral geniculate nucleus can be placed above the surface of the cortex on the side of the pia, rather than below the white matter, and the fibers from it will still go to layer IV. This strongly suggests that there are molecular cues that attract the afferent fibers.

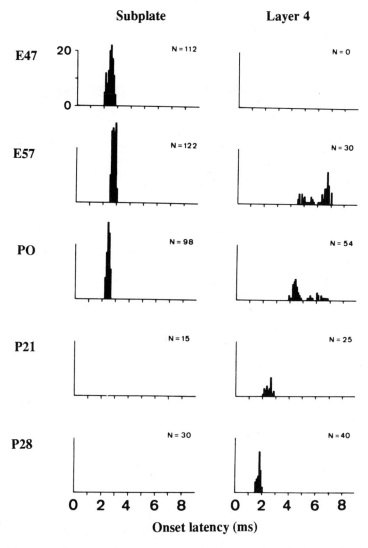

Subplate **Layer 4**

Onset latency (ms)

FIG. 4.5. Monosynaptic connections are found between lateral geniculate and subplate before birth, and between lateral geniculate and layer IV after birth in the cat. Figure shows the latency in subplate and layer IV from stimulation of lateral geniculate at various ages. A latency of around 2 msec represents monosynaptic input; around 4 msec, disynaptic or more. The connection to layer IV becomes monosynaptic between P0 and P21. Reprinted with permission from Friauf and Shatz (1991).

The organization of the layers is disturbed in the reeler mutant mouse (Caviness, 1976). The polymorphic cells of layer VI are found just below the pia. Pyramidal cells are found in an inverted location, with the large ones that are normally in layer V above the small ones that are normally in layers II and III. In spite of being in the wrong layer, the cells make the correct connections and have the correct receptive field properties (Lemmon and Pearlman, 1981). This also shows that there is some factor intrinsic to the cells in layer V, and

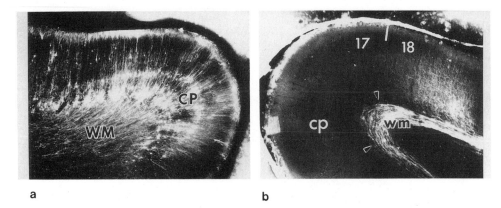

a   b

FIG. 4.6. Lateral geniculate axons do not innervate the cortex if the subplate is missing. (a) Lateral geniculate axons innervating the cortex at P2. (b) Lateral geniculate axons bypassing the cortex at P5 after lesions of the subplate. Reprinted with permission from Ghosh *et al.*, 1990, Requirement for subplate neurons in the formation of thalamocortical connections, *Nature* **347**:179–181. Copyright 1990, MacMillan Magazines Limited.

another factor intrinsic to the cells in layers II and III that enables them to recognize their targets, independent of whether they are located in a normal or abnormal position in the cortex.

Connections within the cortex that project from one layer to another are also specific from the earliest time that they are made. Cells in layer IV develop axons to layer V, which are complete at P15, and to layer II/III, which are

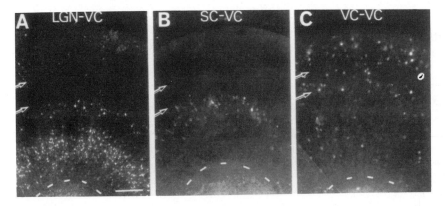

FIG. 4.7. Cells in the visual cortex establish appropriate connections when slices of visual cortex are put into coculture with slices of areas to which the visual cortex normally connects. Label is added to the target, and transported retrogradely back to the cell of origin. When visual cortex is cocultured with lateral geniculate (LGN-VC), cells in layer VI are labeled (A); when cocultured with superior colliculus (SC-VC), cells in layer V are labeled (B); when cocultured with visual cortex (VC-VC), cells in layer II are labeled (C). Arrows mark layer IV. Reprinted with kind permission from Toyama, K., Komatsu, Y., Yamamoto, N., and Kurotani, T., 1993, In vitro studies of visual cortical development and plasticity, *Prog. Neurobiol.* **41**:543–563. Copyright 1992, Elsevier Science, Ltd., The Boulevard, Langford Lane, Kidlington OX5 1GB, UK.

complete at P33 (Callaway and Katz, 1992). Cells in layers II and III project to layer V, passing through layer IV on the way, from the first week onward (Katz, 1991). Thus, some property of the neurons determines that their target is layer V, rather than layer IV.

The topographic organization of afferents from the retina to the lateral geniculate nucleus, and from the lateral geniculate nucleus to the visual cortex, is correctly determined at a coarse level when the afferents first come in (Henderson and Blakemore, 1986; Payne *et al.*, 1988). Unfortunately, the anatomical techniques used to demonstrate this point are not capable of high resolution, and cannot test the fine tuning of the projection very well. Nevertheless, work in the hamster suggests that some fine tuning does take place after the initial connections are made (Naegele *et al.*, 1988). Work on the formation of the map in the rat superior colliculus suggests that this fine tuning is under the control of activity (Simon *et al.*, 1992).

Each set of projections needs a variety of cues to find its way to its target. As an example, consider the projections from the lateral geniculate nucleus to the visual cortex. First, the fibers have to find their way past various other nuclei in the midbrain. When they reach the cortex, they have to stop in the correct area, guided by the subplate neurons. They have to form an approximate topographic map. This could occur simply because neighboring fibers from the lateral geniculate stay together, although there is an inversion of the map along one axis, but not along the perpendicular axis (Nelson and LeVay, 1985). Perhaps the subplate neurons also play a role in topographic organization, but an experiment to test this has not yet been done. Finally they have to stop in the correct layer in the cortex—layer IV. We do not know for certain if this is related to attractive cues in layer IV, or repulsive cues in other layers, but the final result is appropriate. Multiple cues are needed for all of this, some in the midbrain, some in the subplate, and some in the cortex itself.

In summary, the organization of long-distance connections, and of layering within the visual cortex, is under the control of genetics and local molecular cues rather than experience. Indeed, it is hard to see how it could be otherwise, because of the way in which processes cross each other in the final system. Some of it could be organized by timing, so that axons generated early go in one direction, and axons generated later go in another direction, but there is simply not enough time in the development of the central nervous system for all of it to be generated that way. While it is clear that molecular cues are essential for establishing the overall pattern of connectivity in the central nervous system, the pattern is still very coarse. As we will see below, other processes, especially electrical activity, are required for the further refinement of connections.

II. Organization under the Control of Sensory Input and Activity

A large number of physiological properties are clearly under the control of sensory input, and they will be dealt with in the next chapter. One property that has a well-demonstrated anatomical basis is ocular dominance; that is, whether the visual response of a cell is dominated by the left eye or the right eye, which depends on the relative strength of the inputs from the two eyes to the cell. The afferents to layer IV of the visual cortex from left and right eyes initially overlap within the layer (Rakic, 1976; LeVay et al., 1978, 1980). By 6 weeks of age, in both macaque monkey and cat, they have segregated into alternate bands dominated by either the left or the right eye (Fig. 4.8). This process does not occur if electrical activity is abolished chemically (Stryker and Harris, 1986).

A similar phenomenon occurs regarding the pattern of layers in the lateral geniculate nucleus. There are three main layers in the cat, and six in the primate. Initially, endings from each eye ramify through all of them, and the layers are not noticeable (Rakic, 1976; Sretavan and Shatz, 1986). Then the layers form as the right eye endings retract from some layers and the left eye endings retract from others (Fig. 4.9). This process also does not occur in the absence of electrical activity (Shatz and Stryker, 1988). Nor does the segregation into the separate

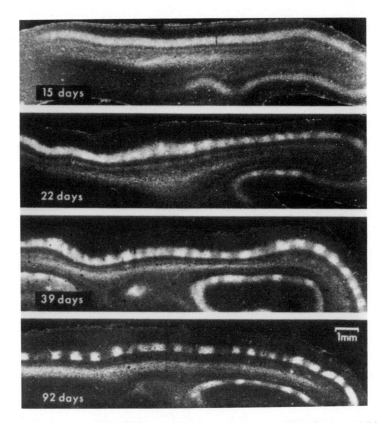

FIG. 4.8. Postnatal development of ocular dominance columns in the visual cortex of the cat. [³H]-Proline was injected into one eye and carried by axoplasmic transport to the visual cortex. The sections are darkfield autoradiographs at four different ages: transported proline shows up as light areas. The sections were horizontal through the visual cortex, with the midline at the top and posterior to the right. At 15 days a continuous band can be seen in layer IV. At 92 days, this band has segregated into clumps representing the label transported from the ipsilateral eye. At 22 and 39 days, intermediate degrees of segregation are seen. Reprinted with permission from LeVay and Stryker (1979).

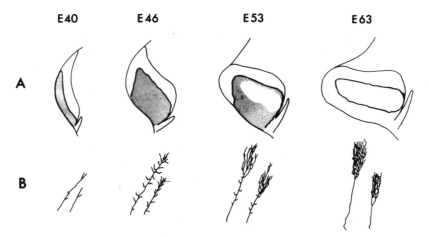

FIG. 4.9. Formation of eye-specific layers in the cat lateral geniculate nucleus. (A) Boundaries of the layers. Shading represents areas where endings from the two eyes overlap. (B) Terminals of representative axons from the retina. Reprinted with permission from Sretavan and Shatz (1986).

ON and OFF pathways discussed in Chapter 2: while single cells in the lateral geniculate of normal kittens respond either at the onset of a stimulus, or at its offset, single cells in the lateral geniculate of kittens that have been reared with no electrical activity respond to both (Dubin et al., 1986).

Within the adult visual cortex, lateral connections are made between columns that deal with like features, for example, horizontal orientation columns to horizontal orientation columns. These connections also are initially widespread (Luhmann et al., 1986; Callaway and Katz, 1990). This process also depends on electrical activity, as shown by experiments where stimulation of the retina is prevented by suturing both eyes shut, and the refinement of columnar connections is consequently abolished (Callaway and Katz, 1991).

How the initial formation of orientation columns occurs is not completely established. Orientation columns are found at birth in the macaque (Wiesel and Hubel, 1974), soon after eye opening in the cat (Hubel and Wiesel, 1963), and not long after eye opening in the ferret (Chapman and Stryker, 1993). Thus, they form in the absence of activity giving information about orientation. There are theories showing that this could occur based on activity patterns generated in the absence of visual information, by competition between ON- and OFF-center inputs (Miller, 1992). Blocking of electrical activity prevents the development of orientation selectivity, if started at P21–23 in the ferret, but does not abolish it altogether (Chapman and Stryker, 1993). Conceivably, orientation specificity could be abolished completely, if electrical activity were blocked even earlier. Consequently, we do not know if orientation columns are like topographic organization, in the sense that there is a basic organization that is refined by activity, or like ocular dominance columns, in the sense that there is little organization in the complete absence of activity.

The properties that can be altered by sensory activity generally involve anatomical changes over fairly short distances, on the order of 1 mm. This is the measure of the width of a few columns in the cortex, or a layer in the lateral geniculate. In many cases, anatomical techniques that will show changes over this distance are not available, or are very hard to employ. Consequently, we cannot give a lot of examples in this chapter, which deals primarily with the anatomy. However, it will become clear that there are numerous examples of physiological reorganizations that can occur when sensory activity is disrupted, and also numerous examples of improvements in psychophysical properties during development, both of which must have an underlying anatomical basis.

III. Events during Differentiation

There are several events that take place in the nervous system after the young neurons have found their way to their final location, and have sent processes out to make connections. One is cell loss through the death of some cells. A second is the pruning or elimination of axon terminals, and in some cases the growth of new ones. A third is the differentiation of the dendrites on the cell. A fourth is the formation and loss of synapses. Each of these occurs during the development of the visual system.

The best documented cell loss occurs among ganglion cells in the retina, and cells in the lateral geniculate nucleus. Major cell loss occurs in the retina between E80 and E120 in the macaque (Rakic and Riley, 1983a) and between E39 and E53 in the cat (Ng and Stone, 1982; Williams et al., 1986). This loss is under genetic control, and is not affected by electrical activity (Friedman and Shatz, 1990). In motor systems, the purpose of cell loss is well established: it matches the number of motoneurons to the number of muscles. In the visual system the purpose is not so clear. Loss of cells in the macaque retina occurs while lamination of the lateral geniculate nucleus is taking place (Fig. 4.10): it

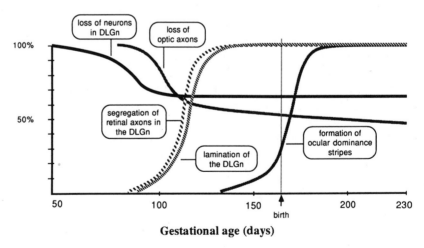

FIG. 4.10. Events in the development of the monkey visual system. DLGn, dorsal lateral geniculate nucleus. Reprinted with permission from Williams, R. W., and Rakic, P., 1988, Elimination of neurons from the rhesus monkey's lateral geniculate nucleus during development, *J. Comp. Neurol.* **272**:424–436. Copyright 1988, John Wiley & Sons, Inc.

can be reduced by taking out the other eye, suggesting a relationship between the cell loss and the elimination of endings from inappropriate layers in the lateral geniculate nucleus (Rakic and Riley, 1983b). However, cell loss in the lateral geniculate nucleus starts at E48, before the retinal fibers arrive, before lamination of the lateral geniculate occurs, and before cortical connections are made (Williams and Rakic, 1988). Matching of nucleus and target therefore does not seem to be the purpose of this loss.

Pruning of axon terminals takes place all over the visual system during development. This is the mechanism whereby ocular dominance columns form in the cortex, and eye-specific layers in the lateral geniculate nucleus. The terminals of retinal ganglion cells in the lateral geniculate initially have side branches in all layers (Fig. 4.9). The side branches in the wrong layers eventually retract (Sretavan and Shatz, 1986). Similarly, the terminals of lateral geniculate cells in layer IV of the visual cortex grow widespread terminals, then some side branches are lost, so that in the adult there are patches of side branches alternating with bare spaces along the axons (LeVay and Stryker, 1979). These alternating areas are the basis for ocular dominance columns in the mature visual system. Likewise, projections to area 18 in the adult cat originate from clusters of cells in area 17. These cells of origin are distributed in bands of uniform density in newborn kittens. The formation of clusters occurs during weeks 2 and 3 by a process of axonal retraction, and possibly also cell death in the deep laminae (Price and Blakemore, 1985).

The right visual cortex, which deals with the left field of view, and the left visual cortex, which deals with the right field of view, are connected through the corpus callosum. The callosum therefore deals primarily with the vertical meridian, which separates the two halves of the field of view. Callosal projections are also widespread early in development, and later retract. In the cat, a wide area of the field of view is connected across the midline to start with, then the area becomes confined to the vertical meridian (Innocenti, 1981), although the initially widespread endings do not penetrate through the cortex to their normal laminar location. In the primate, callosal fibers join secondary visual cortex, but not primary visual cortex. However, the same process of retraction takes place, as well as some elimination of axons (Dehay et al., 1988; LaMantia and Rakic, 1990).

Normally the cells that project from the retina to the lateral geniculate are different from those that project to the superior colliculus. X cells, also known as β cells, which are responsible for fine acuity, project to the lateral geniculate nucleus but not the superior colliculus in the adult cat. At E38 to E43, the proportion of these cells projecting to the superior colliculus is much higher than in the adult (Ramoa et al., 1989). The projections that are not functional in the adult are eliminated by a process that must include elimination of axons to the superior colliculus, because it occurs after the period of cell death is over.

There is also sculpting of the efferent connections of the cortex. Layer V cells in the adult project to the superior colliculus. During development they also project to the spinal cord, which is a natural target for layer V cells from the motor cortex. There is some molecular specificity, because they do not project to the cerebellum, or many other parts of the brain that they pass along the way. At the same time there is a target specificity, which occurs by pruning after the initial projections are made. The cells in the visual cortex eventually lose their projections to the spinal cord (Stanfield and O'Leary, 1985).

The dendrites of cells, like the axons, develop by a process of proliferation and retraction. There are three stages in the development of dendrites after their initial growth (Lund et al., 1977). First, the dendrites grow hairlike processes while the axons are still ramifying. Then, all cells grow a dense set of spines on the dendrites, including those cells that do not have spines in the adult. Then the spines retract, until the adult stage is reached (Fig. 4.11). These stages may occur at different times in different cells, but the same general sequence occurs in all cells (Meyer and Ferres-Torres, 1984).

Synapses are also produced in greater numbers than found in the adult, as one might expect from the overproduction of cells, axons, and dendrites. The first synapses are found in layer I and the subplate, and those on cell bodies, of course, disappear as the cells disappear (Molliver et al., 1973). In the cat there is a rapid increase of synapses between P8 and P37 (Cragg, 1975). Only 1% of synapses are present at birth. The number peaks at 4 to 8 weeks of age, then declines, in all layers (Winfield, 1983). There may be a considerable turnover of synapses during the peak of the period of rearrangements, at 4–6 weeks of age, but there is no marker that can be used to detect this accurately at the present time. A similar situation occurs in the macaque (Bourgeois and Rakic, 1993).

It seems likely that all of these processes, except cell loss, are involved in sensory-dependent plasticity because of the time at which they occur. Both pruning of axon terminals and differentiation of dendrites are postnatal events,

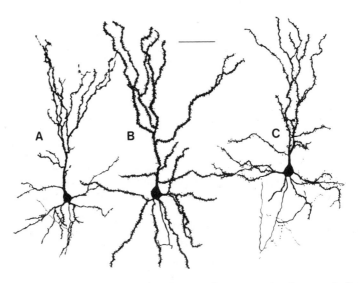

FIG. 4.11. Maturation of pyramidal cells from layer II of macaque visual cortex. Individual cells were stained with the Golgi technique. Typical cells are shown for three ages: (A) at birth; (B) 8 weeks postnatal; (C) adult. Reprinted with permission from Lund, J. S., Boothe, R. G., and Lund, R. D., 1977, Development of neurons in the visual cortex (area 17) of the monkey (Macaca nemestrina): A Golgi study from fetal day 127 to postnatal maturity, *J. Comp. Neurol.* **176:**149–187. Copyright 1977, John Wiley & Sons, Inc.

occurring after the eyes open and while physiological changes are taking place. The number of synapses peaks at the time when the system is most susceptible to sensory-dependent effects. We will discuss how these processes are involved, after giving details of sensory-dependent plasticity.

IV. Summary

The initial events in the development of the visual system, which occur before the connections are formed, are under genetic and molecular control. These include the generation and migration of cells, the projection of their axons to their targets, the general organization of the terminals within the targets, and the specificity of layers within the cortex, including the specificity of afferent connections, efferent connections, and connections within the cortex. Most of this takes place before birth. Later events, occurring after the connections are formed, and in most cases after the eyes open, are under the control of electrical activity. This includes the refinement of maps within a nucleus, the formation of columns within the cortex, and the formation of layers within the lateral geniculate nucleus.

References

Austin, C. P., and Cepko, C. L., 1990, Cellular migration patterns in the developing mouse cerebral cortex, *Development* **110:**713–732.

Blakemore, C., and Molnar, Z., 1990, Factors involved in the establishment of specific interconnections between thalamus and cerebral cortex, *Cold Spring Harbor Symp. Quant. Biol.* **55:**491–504.

Bourgeois, J. P., and Rakic, P., 1993, Changes of synaptic density in the primary visual cortex of the macaque monkey from fetal to adult stage, *J. Neurosci.* **13:**2801–2820.

Callaway, E. M., and Katz, L. C., 1990, Emergence and refinement of clustered horizontal connections in cat striate cortex, *J. Neurosci.* **10:**1134–1153.

Callaway, E. M., and Katz, L. C., 1991, Effects of binocular deprivation on the development of clustered horizontal connections in cat striate cortex, *Proc. Natl. Acad. Sci. USA* **88:**745–749.

Callaway, E. M., and Katz, L. C., 1992, Development of axonal arbors of layer 4 spiny stellate neurons in cat striate cortex, *J. Neurosci.* **12:**570–582.

Caviness, V. S., 1976, Patterns of cell and fiber distribution in the neocortex of the reeler mutant mouse, *J. Comp. Neurol.* **170:**435–448.

Chapman, B., and Stryker, M. P., 1993, Development of orientation selectivity in ferret visual cortex and effects of deprivation, *J. Neurosci.* **13:**5251–5262.

Chun, J. J. M., and Shatz, C. J., 1989, Interstitial cells of the adult neocortical white matter are the remnant of the early generated subplate neuron population, *J. Comp. Neurol.* **282:**555–569.

Cragg, B. G., 1975, The development of synapses in the visual system of the cat, *J. Comp. Neurol.* **160:**147–166.

Dehay, C., Kennedy, H., Bullier, J., and Berland, M., 1988, Absence of interhemispheric connections of area 17 during development in the monkey, *Nature* **331:**348–350.

Dubin, M. W., Stark, L. A., and Archer, S. M., 1986, A role for action-potential activity in the development of neuronal connections in the kitten retinogeniculate pathway, *J. Neurosci.* **6:**1021–1036.

Friauf, E., and Shatz, C. J., 1991, Changing patterns of synaptic input to subplate and cortical plate during development of visual cortex, *J. Neurophysiol.* **66:**2059–2071.

Friauf, E., McConnell, S. K., and Shatz, C. J., 1990, Functional synaptic circuits in the subplate during fetal and early postnatal development of cat visual cortex, *J. Neurosci.* **10:**2601–2613.

Friedman, S., and Shatz, C. J., 1990, The effects of prenatal intracranial infusion of tetrodotoxin on naturally occurring retinal ganglion cell death and optic nerve ultrastructure, *Eur. J. Neurosci.* **2**:243–253.

Ghosh, A., Antonini, A., McConnell, S. K., and Shatz, C. J., 1990, Requirement for subplate neurons in the formation of thalamocortical connections, *Nature* **347**:179–181.

Guillery, R. W., 1974, Visual pathways in albinos, *Sci. Am.* **230(5)**:44–54.

Henderson, Z., and Blakemore, C., 1986, Organization of the visual pathways in the newborn kitten, *Neurosci. Res.* **3**:628–659.

Hubel, D. H., and Wiesel, T. N., 1963, Receptive fields of cells in striate cortex of very young, visually inexperienced kittens, *J. Neurophysiol.* **26**:994–1002.

Innocenti, G. M., 1981, Growth and reshaping of axons in the establishment of visual callosal connections, *Science* **212**:824–827.

Katz, L. C., 1991, Specificity in the development of vertical connections in cat striate cortex, *Eur. J. Neurosci.* **3**:1–9.

Kostovic, I., and Rakic, P., 1990, Developmental history of the transient subplate zone in the visual and somatosensory cortex of the macaque monkey and human brain, *J. Comp. Neurol.* **297**:441–470.

LaMantia, A. S., and Rakic, P., 1990, Axon overproduction and elimination in the corpus callosum of the developing rhesus monkey, *J. Neurosci.* **10**:2156–2175.

LaVail, M. M., Rapaport, D. H., and Rakic, P., 1991, Cytogenesis in the monkey retina, *J. Comp. Neurol.* **309**:86–114.

Lemmon, V., and Pearlman, A. L., 1981, Does laminar position determine the receptive field properties of cortical neurons? A study of corticotectal cells in area 17 of the normal mouse and the reeler mutant, *J. Neurosci.* **1**:83–93.

LeVay, S., and Stryker, M. P., 1979, The development of ocular dominance columns in the cat, *Soc. Neurosci. Symp.* **4**:83–98.

LeVay, S., Stryker, M. P., and Shatz, C. J., 1978, Ocular dominance columns and their development in layer IV of the cat's visual cortex: A quantitative study, *J. Comp. Neurol.* **179**:223–244.

LeVay, S., Wiesel, T. N., and Hubel, D. H., 1980, The development of ocular dominance columns in normal and visually deprived monkeys, *J. Comp. Neurol.* **191**:1–51.

Lorente de Nó, R., 1938, Cerebral cortex: Architectonics, intracortical connections, in: *Physiology of the Nervous System* (J. F. Fulton, ed.), Oxford University Press, London, pp. 288–313.

Luhmann, H. J., Millan, L. M., and Singer, W., 1986, Development of horizontal intrinsic connections in cat striate cortex, *Exp. Brain Res.* **63**:443–448.

Lund, J. S., Boothe, R. G., and Lund, R. D., 1977, Development of neurons in the visual cortex (area 17) of the monkey (Macaca nemestrina): A Golgi study from fetal day 127 to postnatal maturity, *J. Comp. Neurol.* **176**:149–187.

Luskin, M. B., and Shatz, C. J., 1985, Neurogenesis of the cat's primary visual cortex, *J. Comp. Neurol.* **242**:611–631.

Marin-Padilla, M., 1971, Early prenatal ontogenesis of the cerebral cortex (neocortex) of the cat (Felis domestica). A Golgi study. I. The primordial neocortical organization, *Z. Anat. Entwicklungsgesch.* **134**:117–145.

Meyer, G., and Ferres-Torres, R., 1984, Postnatal maturation of nonpyramidal neurons in the visual cortex of the cat, *J. Comp. Neurol.* **228**:226–244.

Miller, K. D., 1992, Development of orientation columns via competition between ON- and OFF-center inputs, *Neuroreport* **3**:73–76.

Molliver, M. E., Kostovic, T., and Van der Loos, H. V., 1973, The development of synapses in cerebral cortex of the human fetus, *Brain Res.* **50**:403–407.

Naegele, J. R., Jhaveri, S., and Schneider, G. E., 1988, Sharpening of topographical projections and maturation of geniculocortical axon arbors in the hamster, *J. Comp. Neurol.* **277**:593–607.

Nelson, S. B., and LeVay, S., 1985, Topographic organization of the optic radiation of the cat, *J. Comp. Neurol.* **240**:322–330.

Ng, A. Y., and Stone, J., 1982, The optic nerve of the cat: Appearance and loss of axons during normal development, *Dev. Brain Res.* **5**:263–271.

Novak, N., and Bolz, J., 1993, Formation of specific efferent connections in organotypic slice cultures from rat visual cortex cocultured with lateral geniculate nucleus and superior colliculus, *Eur. J. Neurosci.* **5**:15–24.

Payne, B. R., Pearson, H. E., and Cornwell, P., 1988, Development of connections in cat visual and auditory cortex, in: *Cerebral Cortex: Development and Maturation of Cerebral Cortex* (A. Peters and E. G. Jones, eds.), Plenum Press, New York, pp. 309–389.

Price, D. J., and Blakemore, C., 1985, Regressive events in the postnatal development of association projections in the visual cortex, *Nature* **316**:721–724.

Rakic, P., 1972, Mode of cell migration to the superficial layers of fetal monkey neocortex, *J. Comp. Neurol.* **145**:61–83.

Rakic, P., 1974, Neurons in rhesus monkey visual cortex: Systematic relation between time of origin and eventual disposition, *Science* **183**:425–427.

Rakic, P., 1976, Prenatal genesis of connections subserving ocular dominance in the rhesus monkey, *Nature* **261**:467–471.

Rakic, P., 1977, Prenatal development of the visual system in rhesus monkey, *Philos. Trans. R. Soc. London Ser. B* **278**:245–260.

Rakic, P., 1992, An overview development of the primate visual system: From photoreceptors to cortical modules, in: *The Visual System from Genesis to Maturity* (R. Lent, ed.), Birkhauser, Boston, pp. 1–17.

Rakic, P., and Riley, K. P., 1983a, Overproduction and elimination of retinal axons in the fetal rhesus monkey, *Science* **219**:1441–1444.

Rakic, P., and Riley, K. P., 1983b, Regulation of axon number in primate optic nerve by prenatal binocular competition, *Nature* **305**:135–137.

Ramoa, A. S., Campbell, G., and Shatz, C. J., 1989, Retinal ganglion β cells project transiently to the superior colliculus during development, *Proc. Natl. Acad. Sci. USA* **86**:2061–2065.

Shatz, C. J., and Luskin, M. B., 1986, The relationship between the geniculocortical afferents and their cortical target cells during development of the cat's primary visual cortex, *J. Neurosci.* **6**:3655–3668.

Shatz, C. J., and Rakic, P., 1981, The genesis of efferent connections from the visual cortex of the fetal rhesus monkey, *J. Comp. Neurol.* **196**:287–307.

Shatz, C. J., and Stryker, M. P., 1988, Prenatal tetrodotoxin infusion blocks segregation of retinogeniculate afferents, *Science* **242**:87–89.

Simon, D. K., Prusky, G. T., O'Leary, D. D. M., and Constantine-Paton, M., 1992, N-methyl-D-aspartate receptor antagonists disrupt the formation of a mammalian neural map, *Proc. Natl. Acad. Sci. USA* **89**:10593–10597.

Sperry, R. W., 1963, Chemoaffinity in the orderly growth of nerve fiber patterns and connections, *Proc. Natl. Acad. Sci. USA* **50**:703–710.

Sretavan, D. W., and Shatz, C. J., 1986, Prenatal development of retinal ganglion cell axons: Segregation into eye-specific layers within the cat's lateral geniculate nucleus, *J. Neurosci.* **6**:234–251.

Stanfield, B. B., and O'Leary, D. D. M., 1985, The transient corticospinal projection from the occipital cortex during the postnatal development of the rat, *J. Comp. Neurol.* **238**:236–248.

Stryker, M. P., and Harris, W. A., 1986, Binocular impulse blockade prevents the formation of ocular dominance columns in cat visual cortex, *J. Neurosci.* **6**:2117–2133.

Toyama, K., Komatsu, Y., Yamamoto, N., and Kurotani, T., 1993, In vitro studies of visual cortical development and plasticity, *Prog. Neurobiol.* **41**:543–563.

Walsh, C., and Cepko, C. L., 1988, Clonally related cortical cells show several migration patterns, *Science* **241**:1342–1345.

Wiesel, T. N., and Hubel, D. H., 1974, Ordered arrangement of orientation columns in monkeys lacking visual experience, *J. Comp. Neurol.* **158**:307–318.

Williams, R. W., and Rakic, P., 1988, Elimination of neurons from the rhesus monkey's lateral geniculate nucleus during development, *J. Comp. Neurol.* **272**:424–436.

Williams, R. W., Bastiani, M. J., Lia, B., and Chalupa, L. M., 1986, Growth cones, dying axons and developmental fluctuations in the fiber population of the cat's optic nerve, *J. Comp. Neurol.* **246**:32–69.

Winfield, D. A., 1983, The postnatal development of synapses in the different laminae of the visual cortex in the normal kitten and in kittens with eyelid suture, *Dev. Brain Res.* **9**:155–169.

Yamamoto, N., Kurotani, T., and Toyama, K., 1989, Neural connections between the lateral geniculate nucleus and visual cortex in vitro, *Science* **245**:192–194.

5

Development of Receptive Field Properties

The physiological properties of most cells in the visual system develop for a period of time after birth. The connections of many cells are not completely formed when the eyes open, and the visual performance of all higher mammals is initially uncertain and groping. Only with use can one analyze the visual image fully and respond to it. There is clearly a learning process occurring. The key questions are: which properties develop, where in the visual system does the development occur, and when does it happen?

Most work on the development of receptive field properties has been done in the cat. The cat is the animal of choice for correlation of receptive field properties with anatomical changes. Unfortunately, cats are hard to work with in behavioral experiments. Monkeys yield more precise results in behavioral studies, but there are not many papers on the development of receptive field properties in this species. Consequently, this chapter will emphasize the cat but give evidence from the monkey wherever possible.

The initial experiments on the development of receptive field properties were prompted by the nature–nurture controversy that was discussed in Chapter 1. At first, authors took somewhat extreme positions. Hubel and Wiesel (1963) were surprised that cells in young kittens respond to the orientation of a bar when it is moved through the receptive field of the cell, that cells with similar orientation sensitivity are located near each other, and that binocular convergence of input from the two eyes onto single cells is like that in the adult. For them, the crucial feature distinguishing cortical cells from lateral geniculate cells was orientation sensitivity, so they emphasized that "much of the richness of visual physiology in the cortex of the adult cat is present in very young kittens without visual experience." They were surprised because vision is poor in kittens at the time of eye opening. Avoidance of objects is not observed until 14 days, and pursuit, following movements, and visual placing appear at 20–25 days (Windle, 1930). Pettigrew (1974), on the other hand, reported that selectivity of cells for disparity improves substantially over the first few weeks. He consequently emphasized the development of receptive field properties after birth. From their different points of view, they were both correct. There is an organization to the properties and location of cells in the visual cortex at birth, and there is also a refinement of those properties resulting from visual experience.

Most studies of receptive field properties in the visual cortex are done in anesthetized, paralyzed animals. This ensures that the eyes will not move, and that a stimulus can be repeated several times so as to give a reliable response. A single cell in the visual cortex is isolated with a microelectrode, then stimuli are projected onto a tangent screen in front of the animal. Since the response of the cell can vary with the length, width, orientation, direction and velocity of movement, color, spatial frequency, and disparity of the object, and there may be interactions between these properties such as movement in depth, it may take several experiments before the properties are fully understood. Three major papers explored the properties of ganglion cells in the cat retina between 1950 and 1974, each one providing a new classification. Since 1968, three major papers have explored the properties of cells in primary visual cortex of the macaque, with numerous details added in the years in between. It seems likely that we now understand the retina, that some new discoveries will be made in primary visual cortex, and that many more experiments will need to be done on the cells in higher visual areas before their properties are fully understood. Consequently, this chapter will not discuss levels of the visual system higher than primary visual cortex.

All authors who have studied receptive fields of cells in the visual cortex in young kittens have noted that the cells are not very responsive. The cells habituate, so that stimuli need to be presented several seconds apart to give the best response, and even then the response is substantially less than in the adult. Close attention needs to be paid to the condition of the animal by monitoring heart rate, blood pressure, and expired CO_2, as a deterioration of these can reduce the specificity of the response even further. However, the susceptibility of young animals to the effects of anesthetic does not account for the lack of specific receptive fields found in well-monitored animals, because cells with receptive fields that are specific for the orientation and direction of movement of the stimulus are found near cells that are not specific for these properties in the same animal under the same conditions.

An important consideration in studying the response of cells in the cat visual system is that the optics are not clear when the eyes open. There is a hyaloid membrane on the posterior surface of the lens (Thorn et al., 1976). This blurs the image on the retina distinctly at 16 days of age, and slightly at 30 days (Bonds and Freeman, 1978). However, for many tasks the effect is not significant, because of the nature of the optical distortions involved. This consideration does not apply to the macaque, where the optical media are clear at birth.

Finally, one needs to emphasize that it is impossible to characterize all aspects of the receptive field of a cell, while also obtaining a substantial sample of cells in a single experiment. This is particularly true when working with young animals. Scientists have tended to concentrate on one aspect of the receptive field of the cell and study it thoroughly. Conclusions have therefore been modified, as scientists attack the same general problem with new and modified stimuli.

I. Development in the Retina and Lateral Geniculate Nucleus

The retina, lateral geniculate nucleus, and visual cortex develop in parallel from an anatomical point of view. So, clearly, maturation of the properties of cells in the cortex will depend on maturation of the properties of cells at lower levels of the system.

An interesting comparison can be made in the monkey between its behavioral response and the responses of cells at various levels of the system by using the contrast sensitivity curve. Contrast sensitivity develops in the monkey over the first year of life (Boothe et al., 1988). Acuity improves, contrast sensitivity improves at all spatial frequencies, and the peak of the curve moves to higher spatial frequency, as it does in the human (Fig. 5.1).

The theoretical limit of spatial resolution imposed by the spacing of the photoreceptors has been calculated by Jacobs and Blakemore (1988) for the monkey. It is called the Nyquist limit, and it increases from 8–10 cycles/degree at 1 week of age to 40–50 cycles/degree in the adult (Fig. 5.2) for the same reasons discussed in Chapter 3 for humans—the photoreceptors move closer together, and the eyeball gets larger. Grating acuity for the most selective neurons in the lateral geniculate is worse than the Nyquist limit at 1 week of age by a factor of 2 (Blakemore and Vital-Durand, 1986), and gets close to the Nyquist limit at around 1 year of age. Cortical neurons are a little worse than lateral geniculate neurons between 10 weeks and 1 year of age. Acuity measured by behavioral tests is worse than the performance of lateral geniculate and cortical neurons by a factor of 2 at 1 week of age, and catches up around 12 weeks of age. Thus, there are some factors located between photoreceptors and lateral geniculate neurons that degrade performance, and others between cortex and behavior

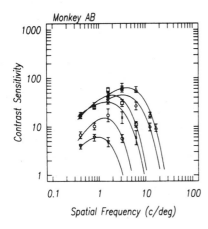 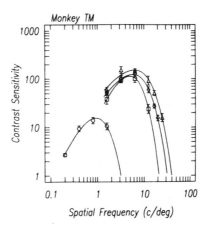

FIG. 5.1. Development of the spatial contrast sensitivity curve for two monkeys. Points for monkey AB taken at 10 (▽), 11 (○), 14 (⊗), 15 (□), 25 (◇), and 38 (△) weeks. Points for monkey TM taken at 5 (○), 12 (□), 20 (◇), and 32 (△) weeks. Reprinted with kind permission from Boothe, R. G., Kiorpes, L., Williams, R. A., and Teller, D., 1988, Operant measurements of spatial contrast sensitivity in infant macaque monkeys during normal development, *Vision Res.* **28**:387–396. Copyright 1988, Elsevier Science, Ltd., The Boulevard, Langford Lane, Kidlington OX5 1GB, UK.

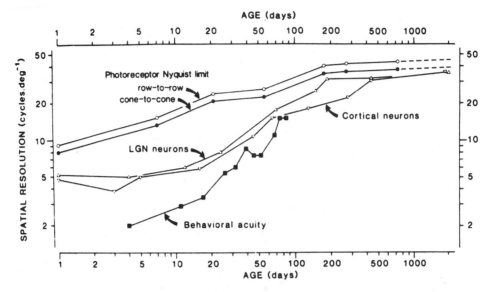

FIG. 5.2. Development of acuity in the monkey measured in behavioral experiments, compared to the capabilities of neurons in the lateral geniculate nucleus and cortex, and the theoretical limit of acuity based on the spacing of photoreceptors. Reprinted with kind permission from Jacobs, D. S., and Blakemore, C., 1988, Factors limiting the postnatal development of visual acuity in the monkey, *Vision Res.* **28:**947–958. Copyright 1988, Elsevier Science, Ltd., The Boulevard, Langford Lane, Kidlington OX5 1GB, UK.

that degrade it further, until the performances at all levels of the system converge around 1 year of age.

A clue as to what some of these degrading factors might be can be obtained from the cat, where the relationship between the anatomy and physiology of the cells involved is more clearly understood. The fine detail cells in the retina of the cat are called X cells when studied physiologically, and β cells when studied anatomically (Boycott and Wassle, 1974). The best spatial frequency for an individual cell is related to the size of the center of the receptive field of the cell, and varies with distance from the center of the retina (Cleland *et al.*, 1979; see Fig. 5.3). There is an absence of cells with very small centers, measured physiologically, during the first 2 weeks of life, corresponding with the poor acuity (Tootle, 1993). However, the anatomical size of β cells in young kittens is small—smaller than in the adult (Rusoff and Dubin, 1978). Consequently, the physiological size of the receptive field exceeds the anatomical size at this age, presumably because of some convergence of lateral excitatory connections within the retina.

The terminal axons of the β cells, in the lateral geniculate nucleus, contract between 3 and 12 weeks of age (Sur *et al.*, 1984). Correspondingly, the spatial resolution of the X cells in the lateral geniculate develops between 3 and 16 weeks of age, in parallel with behavioral measurements, and measurements of the visually evoked response from the cortex (Ikeda and Tremain, 1978). Lateral inhibition producing the surround of the receptive field of cells in the retina matures over the first 4–5 weeks (Rusoff and Dubin, 1977; Hamasaki and Flynn,

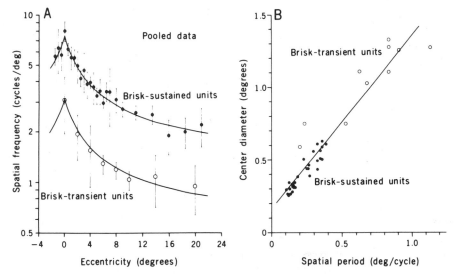

FIG. 5.3. (A) Highest spatial frequency that can be detected, measured with a drifting grating for individual ganglion cells. Results plotted for X (brisk-sustained) cells and Y (brisk-transient) cells, as a function of distance from the center of the retina (eccentricity). (B) Highest detectable spatial frequency is linearly related to the diameter of the center of the receptive field, measured with a bar moved slowly across the receptive field. Reprinted with permission from Cleland, B. G., Harding, T. H., and Tulunay-Keesey, U., 1979, Visual resolution and receptive field size: Examination of two kinds of cat retinal ganglion cells, *Science* **205**:1015–1017. Copyright 1979, American Association for the Advancement of Science.

1977). This occurs in parallel with the development of the center of the receptive field (Tootle, 1993). The additional lateral inhibition that occurs in the lateral geniculate nucleus is immature at 4 weeks of age (Tootle and Friedlander, 1986) and matures after that. As lateral inhibition at both of these levels develops, contrast sensitivity at low frequencies compared to contrast sensitivity at the peak of the contrast sensitivity curve (low-frequency falloff) decreases correspondingly.

Y cells are primarily responsible for detection of movement. Their temporal resolution, measured in the lateral geniculate, improves substantially between 2 and 8 weeks of age, and a little more after that (Wilson *et al.*, 1982). It is difficult to distinguish Y cells from X cells in 3-week-old kittens (Rusoff and Dubin, 1977; Daniels *et al.*, 1978). However, their morphological counterparts, α and β cells, can be distinguished from each other at this age by anatomical criteria (Tootle, 1993). Thus, the distinction between X and Y cells is conferred by synaptic mechanisms that develop after the anatomy is established. The spatial resolution of Y cells in the lateral geniculate decreases with age (Tootle and Friedlander, 1989), probably because the terminal arbors in the lateral geniculate nucleus of α cells from the retina expand between 3 and 12 weeks of age (Sur *et al.*, 1984).

The conclusion is that the development of acuity and the low-frequency falloff in the contrast sensitivity curve depend on processing beyond the photoreceptors as well as on the development of the photoreceptors, just as predicted to be the case for humans (Banks and Bennett, 1988). Changes in the physiological properties of cells in the retina, as well as in the size of their terminal arborizations in the lateral geniculate contribute to changes in acuity. Changes in lateral inhibitory mechanisms in both retina and lateral geniculate contribute to low-frequency falloff. There are also additional factors in the cortex, suggested by the comparison studied by Jacobs and Blakemore (1988), but these have not been specifically identified.

II. Development in the Visual Cortex

The properties of cortical cells in the cat that depend particularly on the retina and lateral geniculate, such as spatial and temporal resolution, develop in parallel with the retina and lateral geniculate. This shows up as an increase in spatial frequency selectivity (Derrington and Fuchs, 1981) and a decrease in the size of the center of the receptive field (Braastad and Heggelund, 1985). In addition, the sensitivity for contrast for a stimulus of the optimal spatial frequency improves dramatically. A contrast of no more than 50% can be detected at 2 weeks of age, while a contrast of 1–3% can be detected at 8 weeks of age (Derrington and Fuchs, 1981).

The proportion of cells that respond to visual stimuli also increases with age, as it does in retina and lateral geniculate. However, more unresponsive cells are found in layers II, III, and V in young animals than in the other layers (Albus and Wolf, 1984). This difference occurs partly because layers II and III are the last to develop anatomically, and partly because layers IV and VI are the ones that receive direct input from the lateral geniculate nucleus, and are therefore the first to get visual input.

The distinguishing physiological features of the visual cortex, as opposed to the lateral geniculate, are selectivity for direction of movement and for orientation; convergence of ON and OFF inputs onto a single cell; convergence of left and right eye inputs onto a single cell; and selectivity for the disparity of the stimulus for binocular cells. One might expect that these would develop with a different time course from retina and lateral geniculate because of the complexity of the stimulus features encoded, but in fact they develop pretty much in parallel.

Some cells specific for the direction of movement of a stimulus are found in the youngest animals recorded from, in the sense that they respond to movement along the preferred axis much better than movement along the axis perpendicular to this (Hubel and Wiesel, 1963; Pettigrew, 1974; Blakemore and Van Sluyters, 1975; see Fig. 5.4). When one considers specificity for the *orientation* of the stimulus, the situation becomes complicated by the definition of exactly what is meant. For cells that respond to stationary stimuli, the situation is clear: one flashes a stimulus on the receptive field in various different orientations, and tests whether the response to one orientation (the preferred orientation) is greater than the response to other orientations. Unfortunately, this test cannot always be applied in young animals, because the rather unresponsive cells that are found often respond fairly clearly to moving stimuli, but not at all clearly to stationary stimuli (Hubel and Wiesel, 1963; Albus and Wolf, 1984).

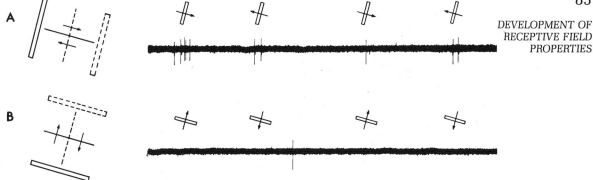

FIG. 5.4. A cell responding to direction of movement from the cortex of an 8-day-old kitten with no previous visual experience. A bar of light, 1° by 5°, was moved across the receptive field of the cell at 5°/sec. On the left is shown the bar in relation to the center of the receptive field, which was in the middle. On the right is shown the train of action potentials, with the movement of the stimulus shown above. The cell responded to a bar moving from 4 o'clock to 10 o'clock and back, but not to a bar moving from 7 o'clock to 1 o'clock and back. Reprinted with permission from the *Journal of Neurophysiology*, Hubel and Wiesel (1963).

When the cell does not respond clearly to stationary stimuli, scientists have measured how the response changes as the stimulus is moved in directions away from the preferred direction. The quantitative measurement of response as a function of the angle of the direction of movement is known as a direction tuning curve (see Fig. 5.5). A direction tuning curve can be measured for movement of a spot and also for movement of a bar. If the curve is narrower for bars than for spots, then this implies that the cell is more specific for the bar than for the spot, and the cell is said to be specific for the orientation of the stimulus, as well as for the direction of movement. There is no doubt that the

FIG. 5.5. Orientation tuning curves produced in a complex cell by light bars of different lengths. The tuning sharpens as the bar is lengthened from 1° (short) to 4° (long). Reprinted with permission from the *Journal of Neurophysiology*, Henry *et al.* (1974).

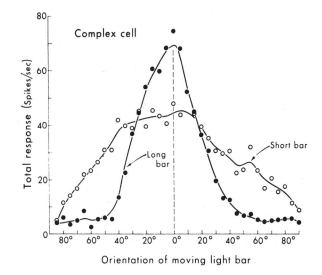

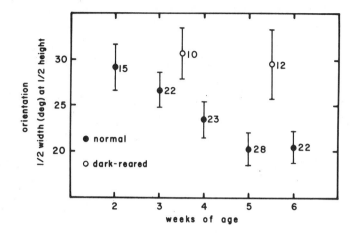

FIG. 5.6. Development of orientation specificity in the visual cortex of the cat. Responses are taken for movement of a stimulus through the receptive field at various orientations, and note taken of the angle at which the response falls to half of the peak response, to give an orientation tuning curve (for an example of such a curve, see Fig. 5.5). The graph represents how far this angle is from the peak, by taking half the angle (¹/₂ width) between the two orientations where the response falls to half the peak (¹/₂ height). Orientation specificity falls from 30° at 2 weeks of age to 20° at 5–6 weeks of age. Note that orientation specificity remains immature if the animal is reared in the dark. Reprinted with permission from Bonds, A. B., 1979, Development of orientation tuning in the visual cortex of kittens, in: *Developmental Neurobiology of Vision*, Plenum Press.

direction tuning curve gets narrower between 2 and 5 weeks of age (Bonds, 1979; see Fig. 5.6). A less time-consuming measurement is to compare the response to the preferred orientation and direction of movement with the response to movement perpendicular to this over a sample of cells. The percentage of cells showing little or no response for movement of a bar perpendicular to the preferred orientation (orientation-selective cells) increases substantially with age (Blakemore and Van Sluyters, 1975; see Fig. 5.7).

The picture is complicated in the cat by the cloudiness of the optics at early ages. This factor does not counter the point that orientation selectivity exists soon after eye opening. However, it may complicate the measurement of the increase in orientation selectivity with age. In the ferret, the optics of the eye are clear, from the time of eye opening, and maturation of orientation selectivity can be more clearly measured (Chapman and Stryker, 1993).

While the selectivity of individual cells for orientation improves with age, the general organization for orientation is established by the time that the eyes open (Fig. 5.8). Cells responding to similar orientations are located near each other in both cat (Hubel and Wiesel, 1963) and monkey (Wiesel and Hubel, 1974).

The maturation of orientation selectivity can also be seen using the 2-deoxyglucose technique. 2-Deoxyglucose is taken up by active cells, but not metabolized, and consequently can be used as a marker of cellular activity. To test orientation selectivity, the animal is stimulated with moving stripes of a particular orientation, then its cortex is assayed for [³H]-2-deoxyglucose taken up by the cells. In the adult, there are patches of cells, demonstrating orientation

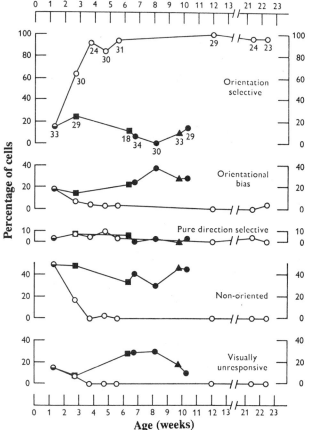

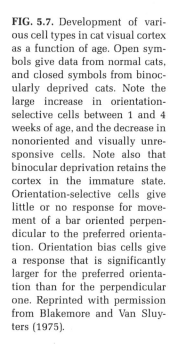

FIG. 5.7. Development of various cell types in cat visual cortex as a function of age. Open symbols give data from normal cats, and closed symbols from binocularly deprived cats. Note the large increase in orientation-selective cells between 1 and 4 weeks of age, and the decrease in nonoriented and visually unresponsive cells. Note also that binocular deprivation retains the cortex in the immature state. Orientation-selective cells give little or no response for movement of a bar oriented perpendicular to the preferred orientation. Orientation bias cells give a response that is significantly larger for the preferred orientation than for the perpendicular one. Reprinted with permission from Blakemore and Van Sluyters (1975).

columns. Before 21 days of age, patchiness is only found in layer IV (Thompson *et al.*, 1983). Between 21 and 35 days of age, the patches mature. As the orientation tuning demonstrated by physiological techniques becomes tighter, the orientation columns demonstrated by anatomical techniques become sharper.

One might expect from the anatomy that binocular convergence would change substantially after birth. As described in Chapter 3, the endings in layer IV of the cortex coming from the lateral geniculate are overlapped at 3 weeks of age, and segregate into eye-specific bands over the next few weeks (LeVay *et al.*, 1978). Consequently, long penetrations in layer IV of 10- to 17-day-old animals show a lot of binocular cells, while similar recordings in adult animals jump from cells driven largely by one eye to cells driven largely by the other. However, there is substantial convergence from the two eyes onto cells in other layers in adult animals, so that this effect is not very noticeable in ocular dominance histograms that include a sample of cells from all layers (Hubel and Wiesel, 1963; Albus and Wolf, 1984; Stryker and Harris, 1986).

One of the first studies on development in the visual cortex dealt with disparity selectivity in the cat (Pettigrew, 1974). This was an excellent choice of subject, given the observation that stereoscopic depth perception, which de-

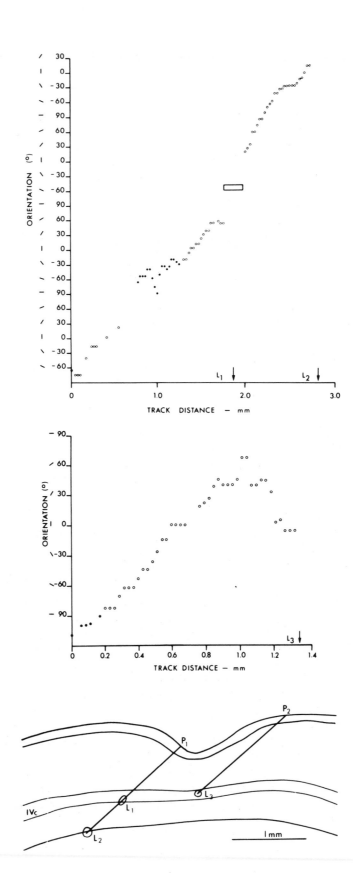

pends on disparity, develops late after birth. Pettigrew found a substantial improvement in disparity selectivity with age, using bars of light as a stimulus (Fig. 5.9). Experiments with gratings (Freeman and Ohzawa, 1992) suggest that the improvement may be largely related to the increase in spatial frequency selectivity of the cells. Unfortunately, similar experiments have not been done in the monkey, which has much better stereoscopic acuity than the cat. Nor do we know anything about the development of cells excited by positive and negative disparity, cells responding to objects nearer than the fixation point, compared to cells responding to objects farther away, and cells inhibited by a specific disparity. This is unfortunate, given that behavioral observations show that stereoscopic vision has a rapid onset that is more clearly defined than any other property in the visual system.

The bulk of these studies have been carried out on primary visual cortex (area 17) in the cat. The three main areas that area 17 projects to in the cat are defined as areas 18, 19, and the lateral suprasylvian gyrus. Studies on cells in area 18 (Blakemore and Price, 1987; Milleret *et al.*, 1988) and the lateral suprasylvian gyrus (Price *et al.*, 1988) give results that are not remarkably different from those in area 17.

III. Development of Receptive Field Properties in the Absence of Light

Early in the history of this field, the nature–nurture controversy prompted the question: what happens to the receptive field properties of cells in the visual cortex in the absence of light? Do they mature, do they remain immature, or do they degenerate?

The initial experiments were done with animals reared in the light with the eyelids of both eyes sutured shut, known as binocular deprivation (Wiesel and Hubel, 1965; Pettigrew, 1974; Singer and Tretter, 1976). Receptive fields were found to be immature, that is, not very specific for the orientation or direction of movement of the stimulus (Fig. 5.7). However, light does reach the retina through closed eyelids, and cells in the visual cortex can detect the direction of movement of a stimulus (Spear *et al.*, 1978), so binocular lid suture does not involve total deprivation.

To avoid all stimulation of the visual system, a better procedure is to rear animals in total darkness. In this case also, the receptive fields of most cells are immature and not very specific for orientation and direction of movement (Blakemore and Van Sluyters, 1975; Buisseret and Imbert, 1976; Cynader *et al.*, 1976; Bonds, 1979; see Fig. 5.6). Sensitivity to the contrast of the stimulus remains low, and the preferred spatial frequency improves up to 3 weeks of age, but not after that (Derrington, 1984). The cells that do retain some specificity for

FIG. 5.8. Two penetrations from the visual cortex of a rhesus monkey with no prior visual experience at 17 days of age. There is a regular progression of orientations as the electrode is advanced at an oblique angle. Reconstruction of the tracks shown at lower right. Reprinted with permission from Wiesel, T. N., and Hubel, D. H., 1974, Ordered arrangement of orientation columns in monkeys lacking visual experience, *J. Comp. Neurol.* **158**:307–318. Copyright 1974, John Wiley & Sons, Inc.

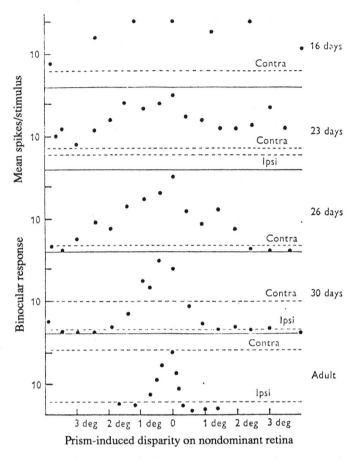

FIG. 5.9. Development of disparity sensitivity in the visual cortex of the cat. Dashed lines give spontaneous activity, circles give response (sometimes inhibition) for various different degrees of disparity. Reprinted with permission from Pettigrew (1974).

orientation tend to be monocularly driven (Blakemore and Van Sluyters, 1975; Leventhal and Hirsch, 1980).

Only one laboratory has made a direct comparison between the effects of dark rearing and binocular deprivation (Mower *et al.*, 1981). The ocular dominance histogram from dark-reared animals was normal, while the histogram from binocularly deprived animals contained more monocular cells. This may occur because the retinas of binocularly deprived animals can detect movement of bright objects (see above) and the stimulation of cells through the two eyes is not concordant, as in strabismus (see Chapter 7). In addition, the binocularly deprived animals had a lot of cells that could not be driven by any visual stimulus, and the dark-reared animals had a lot of cells that could be driven by all orientations and directions of movement. In both cases there were few cells specific for orientation and direction of movement of the stimulus. Thus, while there are differences between the two procedures, because of the fact that there is some visual stimulation in binocular deprivation and none in dark rearing, the final result from both procedures is a cortex with few physiologically normal cells.

One can compare the receptive fields of cells in dark-reared animals with normal animals of the same age. There is some improvement in specificity of the receptive fields up to 3–5 weeks of age in both light-reared and dark-reared animals (Buisseret and Imbert, 1976; Derrington, 1984), followed by a loss of specificity after that in the dark-reared ones. So the answer to the nature–nurture question, as so often happens in biology, is not either–or, but both. There is maturation of receptive field properties in visually inexperienced animals over the first few weeks, some degeneration after that, and the final result is that the receptive fields are immature.

Experiments on dark-reared animals are complicated by an important point that has not yet been analyzed. Rearing in the dark leads to disruption of the day–night cycle, and disturbances in the levels of circulating hormones, particularly melatonin and the adrenal hormones (Evered and Clark, 1985). Morphological effects, such as a reduction in the thickness of the cortex, are found in all parts of cortex in dark-reared animals. Are the results found in the visual cortex in dark-reared animals related to changes in the activity in the afferent fibers, or to more general hormonal changes? Unfortunately, with one or two exceptions (Aoki and Siekevitz, 1985; Daw, 1986) nobody has studied this question by comparing effects on the visual system with effects on other systems. It seems likely that there are both direct and indirect effects.

What are the mechanisms that cause the receptive fields of cells in dark-reared animals to lose their orientation and direction selectivity? There are few anatomical differences between light- and dark-reared animals. The number of cells under 1 mm^2 of cortical surface remains normal. There is a delay in the development of the number of synapses, but the effect is not large (Winfield, 1983). The cortex is thinner, and this reflects a decrease in the amount of neuropil, but which element of the neuropil is not clear (Takacs et al., 1992). On the positive side, there is a decrease in the extent of the basal dendrites in pyramidal cells at the border of layers II and IV in dark-reared animals (Reid and Daw, 1995).

Some scientists predict there should be a difference in the physiology of the inhibitory GABA system, because the orientation and direction specificity of cells is at least partly related to inhibitory mechanisms in the adult (Sillito, 1984). There may be a reduction, or a delay in the development of the number of symmetric synapses, which are the inhibitory synapses (Winfield, 1983; Gabbott and Stewart, 1987). However, the percentage of cells that contain GABA and the parameters of binding to GABA receptors are the same in normal and dark-reared animals (Mower et al., 1988). Moreover, GABA mechanisms can clearly be shown to be present in dark-reared animals (Tanaka et al., 1987; Tsumoto and Freeman, 1987). Consequently, no clear mechanism has yet been found to account for the physiological and functional changes found in dark-reared animals.

IV. Summary

This work can be summarized as follows: some elements of the organization of the visual system are present at birth; there is very substantial development over the first 4 weeks of postnatal life in parallel with the large increase in the number of synapses during this period; and there is a further refinement of properties over the next 3 months or so. These ages apply to the cat, and are different in the primate, but the same general sequence of events occurs in both species.

The elements of a system of orientation columns are present at birth, but the selectivity of individual cells within this system of columns develops after birth. Some cells are responsive to direction of movement at birth. On the other hand, the input from the two eyes to the cortex is initially overlapped, and only segregates into eye-specific columns after birth. Sensitivity to disparity develops over the same period as segregation of ocular dominance. Acuity improves as the size of the center of the receptive fields of the sustained cells gets smaller, and the eyeball gets larger. Movement sensitivity improves as the temporal properties of the Y cell system improve.

The development of physiological properties therefore tallies with the development of psychophysical properties. In both cases, most properties, with the exception of stereopsis, exist at birth, but substantial refinement and tuning occurs postnatally.

References

Albus, K., and Wolf, W., 1984, Early postnatal development of neuronal function in the kitten's visual cortex: A laminar analysis, J. Physiol. (London) **348**:153–185.

Aoki, C., and Siekevitz, P., 1985, Ontogenetic changes in the cyclic adenosine 3',5'-monophosphate-stimulable phosphorylation of cat visual cortex proteins, particularly of microtubule-associated protein 2 (MAP 2): Effects of normal and dark rearing and of the exposure to light, J. Neurosci. **5**:2465–2483.

Banks, M. S., and Bennett, P. J., 1988, Optical and photoreceptor immaturities limit the spatial and chromatic vision of human neonates, J. Opt. Soc. Am. [A] **5**:2059–2079.

Blakemore, C., and Price, D. J., 1987, The organization and post-natal development of area 18 of the cat's visual cortex, J. Physiol. (London) **384**:263–292.

Blakemore, C., and Van Sluyters, R. C., 1975, Innate and environmental factors in the development of the kitten's visual cortex, J. Physiol. (London) **248**:663–716.

Blakemore, C., and Vital-Durand, F., 1986, Organization and post-natal development of the monkey's lateral geniculate nucleus, J. Physiol. (London) **380**:453–491.

Bonds, A. B., 1979, Development of orientation tuning in the visual cortex of kittens, in: Developmental Neurobiology of Vision (R. D. Freeman, ed.), Plenum Press, New York, pp. 31–41.

Bonds, A. B., and Freeman, R. D., 1978, Development of optical quality in the kitten eye, Vision Res. **18**:391–398.

Boothe, R. G., Kiorpes, L., Williams, R. A., and Teller, D., 1988, Operant measurements of spatial contrast sensitivity in infant macaque monkeys during normal development, Vision Res. **28**:387–396.

Boycott, B. B., and Wassle, H., 1974, The morphological type of ganglion cells of the domestic cat's retina, J. Physiol. (London) **240**:397–419.

Braastad, B. O., and Heggelund, P., 1985, Development of spatial receptive field organization and orientation selectivity in kitten striate cortex, J. Neurophysiol. **53**:1158–1178.

Buisseret, P., and Imbert, M., 1976, Visual cortical cells: Their developmental properties in normal and dark-reared kittens, J. Physiol. (London) **255**:511–525.

Chapman, B., and Stryker, M. P., 1993, Development of orientation selectivity in ferret visual cortex and effects of deprivation, J. Neurosci. **13**:5251–5262.

Cleland, B. G., Harding, T. H., and Tulunay-Keesey, U., 1979, Visual resolution and receptive field size: Examination of two kinds of cat retinal ganglion cell, Science **205**:1015–1017.

Cynader, M., Berman, N., and Hein, A., 1976, Recovery of function in cat visual cortex following prolonged deprivation, Exp. Brain Res. **25**:139–156.

Daniels, J. D., Pettigrew, J. D., and Norman, J. L., 1978, Development of single-neuron responses in kitten's lateral geniculate nucleus, *J. Neurophysiol.* **41**:1373–1393.

Daw, N. W., 1986, Effect of dark rearing on development of myelination in cat visual cortex, *Soc. Neurosci. Abstr.* **12**:785.

Derrington, A. M., 1984, Development of spatial frequency selectivity in striate cortex of vision-deprived cats, *Exp. Brain Res.* **55**:431–437.

Derrington, A. M., and Fuchs, A. F., 1981, The development of spatial-frequency selectivity in kitten striate cortex, *J. Physiol. (London)* **316**:1–10.

Evered, D., and Clark, S., 1985, *Photoperiodism, Melatonin and the Pineal*, Pitman, London.

Freeman, R. D., and Ohzawa, I., 1992, Development of binocular vision in the kitten's striate cortex, *J. Neurosci.* **12**:4721–4736.

Gabbott, P. C. A., and Stewart, M. G., 1987, Quantitative morphological effects of dark rearing and light exposure on the synaptic connectivity of layer 4 in the rat visual cortex (area 17), *Exp. Brain Res.* **68**:103–114.

Hamasaki, D. I., and Flynn, J. T., 1977, Physiological properties of retinal ganglion cells of 3-week-old kittens, *Vision Res.* **17**:275–284.

Henry, G. L., Dreher, B., and Bishop, P. O., 1974, Orientation specificity of cells in cat striate cortex, *J. Neurophysiol.* **37**:1394–1409.

Hubel, D. H., and Wiesel, T. N., 1963, Receptive fields of cells in striate cortex of very young, visually inexperienced kittens, *J. Neurophysiol.* **26**:994–1002.

Ikeda, I., and Tremain, K. E., 1978, The development of spatial resolving power of lateral geniculate neurones in kitten, *Exp. Brain Res.* **31**:193–206.

Jacobs, D. S., and Blakemore, C., 1988, Factors limiting the postnatal development of visual acuity in the monkey, *Vision Res.* **28**:947–958.

LeVay, S., Stryker, M. P., and Shatz, C. J., 1978, Ocular dominance columns and their development in layer IV of the cat's visual cortex: A quantitative study, *J. Comp. Neurol.* **179**:223–244.

Leventhal, A. G., and Hirsch, H. V. B., 1980, Receptive-field properties of different classes of neurons in visual cortex of normal and dark-reared cats, *J. Neurophysiol.* **43**:111–1132.

Milleret, C., Gary-Bobo, E., and Buisseret, P., 1988, Comparative development of cell properties in cortical area 18 of normal and dark-reared kittens, *Exp. Brain Res.* **71**:8–20.

Mower, G. D., Berry, D., Burchfiel, J. L., and Duffy, F. H., 1981, Comparison of the effects of dark rearing and binocular suture on development and plasticity of cat visual cortex, *Brain Res.* **220**:255–267.

Mower, G. D., Rustad, R., and White, W. F., 1988, Quantitative comparisons of gamma-aminobutyric acid neurons and receptors in the visual cortex of normal and dark-reared cats, *J. Comp. Neurol.* **272**:293–302.

Pettigrew, J. D., 1974, The effect of visual experience on the development of stimulus specificity by kitten cortical neurones, *J. Physiol. (London)* **237**:49–74.

Price, D. J., Zumbroich, T. J., and Blakemore, C., 1988, Development of stimulus selectivity and functional organisation in the suprasylvian visual cortex of the cat, *Proc. R. Soc. London Ser. B* **233**:123–163.

Reid, S. N. M., and Daw, N. W., 1995, Dark-rearing changes microtubule-associated protein 2 (MAP 2) dendrites but not subplate neurons in cat visual cortex, *J. Comp. Neurol.* **355**:470–478.

Rusoff, A. C., and Dubin, M. W., 1977, Development of receptive field properties of retinal ganglion cells in kittens, *J. Neurophysiol.* **40**:1188–1198.

Rusoff, A. C., and Dubin, M. W., 1978, Kitten ganglion cells: Dendritic field size at 3 weeks of age and correlation with receptive field size, *Invest. Ophthalmol. Vis. Sci.* **17**:819–821.

Sherk, H., and Stryker, M. P., 1976, Quantitative study of cortical orientation selectivity in visually inexperienced kitten, *J. Neurophysiol.* **39**:63–70.

Sherman, S. M., 1972, Development of interocular alignment in cats, *Brain Res.* **37**:187–203.

Sillito, A. M., 1984, Functional considerations of the operation of GABAergic inhibitory processes in the visual cortex, in: *Cerebral Cortex* (E. G. Jones and A. Peters, eds.), Plenum Press, New York, pp. 91–117.

Singer, W., and Tretter, F., 1976, Receptive field properties and neuronal connectivity in striate and parastriate cortex of contour-deprived cats, *J. Neurophysiol.* **39**:613–630.

Spear, P. D., Tong, L., and Langsetmo, A., 1978, Striate cortex neurons of binocularly deprived kittens respond to visual stimuli through the closed eyelids, *Brain Res.* **155**:141–146.

Stryker, M. P., and Harris, W. A., 1986, Binocular impulse blockade prevents the formation of ocular dominance columns in cat visual cortex, *J. Neurosci.* **6:**2117–2133.

Sur, M., Weller, R. E., and Sherman, S. M., 1984, Development of X- and Y-cell retinogeniculate terminations in kittens, *Nature* **310:**246–249.

Takacs, J., Saillour, P., Imbert, M., Bogner, M., and Hamori, J., 1992, Effect of dark rearing on the volume of visual cortex (areas 17 and 18) and the number of visual cortical cells in young kittens, *J. Neurosci. Res.* **32:**449–459.

Tanaka, K., Freeman, R. D., and Ramoa, A. S., 1987, Dark-reared kittens: GABA sensitivity of cells in the visual cortex, *Exp. Brain Res.* **65:**673–675.

Thompson, I. D., Kossut, M., and Blakemore, C., 1983, Development of orientation columns in cat striate cortex revealed by 2-deoxyglucose autoradiography, *Nature* **301:**712–715.

Thorn, F., Gollender, M., and Erickson, P., 1976, The development of the kitten's visual optics, *Vision Res.* **16:**1145–1149.

Tootle, J. S., 1993, Early postnatal development of visual function in ganglion cells of the cat retina, *J. Neurophysiol.* **69:**1645–1660.

Tootle, J. S., and Friedlander, M. J., 1986, Postnatal development of receptive field surround inhibition in kitten dorsal lateral geniculate nucleus, *J. Neurophysiol.* **56:**523–541.

Tootle, J. S., and Friedlander, M. J., 1989, Postnatal development of the spatial contrast sensitivity of X- and Y-cells in the kitten retinogeniculate pathway, *J. Neurosci.* **9:**1325–1340.

Tsumoto, T., and Freeman, R. D., 1987, Dark-reared cats: Responsivity of cortical cells influenced pharmacologically by an inhibitory antagonist, *Exp. Brain Res.* **65:**666–672.

Wiesel, T. N., and Hubel, D. H., 1965, Comparison of the effects of unilateral and bilateral eye closure on cortical unit responses in kittens, *J. Neurophysiol.* **28:**1029–1040.

Wiesel, T. N., and Hubel, D. H., 1974, Ordered arrangement of orientation columns in monkeys lacking visual experience, *J. Comp. Neurol.* **158:**307–318.

Wilson, J. R., Tessin, D. E., and Sherman, S. M., 1982, Development of the electrophysiological properties of Y-cells in the kitten's medial interlaminar nucleus, *J. Neurosci.* **2:**562–571.

Windle, W. F., 1930, Normal behavioral reactions of kittens correlated with the postnatal development of nerve-fiber density in the spinal gray matter, *J. Comp. Neurol.* **50:**479–497.

Winfield, D. A., 1983, The postnatal development of synapses in the different laminae of the visual cortex in the normal kitten and in kittens with eyelid suture, *Dev. Brain Res.* **9:**155–169.

II

Amblyopia and the Effects of Visual Deprivation

6

Modifications to the Visual Input That Lead to Nervous System Changes

Early in life, any optical or motor deficit that produces a degradation of the image on the retina can lead to changes in the visual cortex that enable the individual to cope with problems from the degradation. Unfortunately, such deficits are all too common. The worst are deficits where the image on the left retina is not coordinated with the image on the right retina. In such cases the visual cortex will receive mismatched signals, and either suppress one image, or change its wiring to try to bring the signals into synchrony with each other. We will briefly describe the deficits found in humans in this chapter. The next chapter considers animal models that describe the behavioral, anatomical, and physiological results of such deficits. Then, we will come back to the nature of the deficits found in humans, and describe them in more detail in the light of the mechanisms that have been discovered. Finally, the concept of a critical period will be discussed, and how the critical period varies with the deficit, and how this can affect the treatment that is used. Deficits found in humans include strabismus, anisometropia, astigmatism, myopia, and cataract.

The general clinical term for the pathology resulting from optical deficits in childhood is *amblyopia*. The literal translation of this Greek word is "blunt sight," and this is a good description. The result is not blindness, but a distortion and muddling of the connections in the cortex. How the connections get rewired clearly depends on the nature of the optical deficit. In all cases there is a loss of acuity, but what amblyopia means beyond that varies with the cause. How amblyopia varies from case to case is a fascinating question that will be discussed after the causes and the anatomical and physiological mechanisms have been described.

I. Strabismus

Strabismus is a deficit in the muscular control of the eyes, so that the eyes look in different directions. One eye may look inward (esotropia) or outward (exotropia), and sometimes upward (hypertropia) or downward (hypotropia). There are numerous causes of strabismus, some being motor and some sensory (von Noorden, 1990.) The causes include paralysis of an eye muscle; mechanical problems in movements of the eye; a poor image on the retina so that there is no good signal for fixation; refractive errors that disrupt the normal relation between focusing and convergence of the eyes; and poor control of eye movements by the central nervous system.

Esotropia is the leading cause of amblyopia in children. Frequently it is associated with hyperopia, where the image in the resting condition is focused behind the retina (Atkinson, 1993). To bring the image into focus, the eye has to accommodate. The eyes tend to converge when they accommodate (Fig. 6.1). This is a useful mechanism in normal vision, designed to keep the image in focus and at the same time have it fall on corresponding parts of the two retinas when looking from a distant object to a near one. The connection between accommodation and convergence is an automatic involuntary one. Thus, hyperopia automatically leads to convergence. Many children are born with hyperopia and their focus becomes normal over time through growth of the eyeball. However, some have high hyperopia which continues until 2–3 years of age because of an abnormally small eyeball, and they tend to become esotropic (Ingram *et al.*, 1986). The continued convergence associated with the hyperopia upsets the mechanism for binocular fusion.

Esotropia may also be associated with an abnormal relationship between accommodation and convergence in individuals who are emmetropic. For some

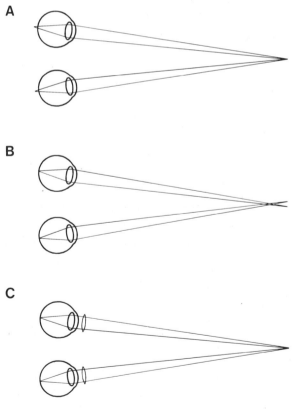

FIG. 6.1. Hyperopia leads to the eyes turning inward. (A) The image is focused behind the retina in the resting state. (B) The act of accommodation, to bring the image into focus, leads to the eyes turning inward, because of the connection between accommodation and convergence. The image will not be in focus for both eyes, but rather will fall on noncorresponding parts of the two retinas. (C) The condition can easily be corrected with spectacles.

people, the amount of convergence associated with accommodation is excessive (this is called a high AC/A ratio). Thus, any attempt to look at a nearby object tends to make the person cross-eyed. This can be overcome by the control of vergence by binocular fusion. In some cases, however, the fusion mechanism is not powerful enough, and the result is esotropia.

Some children are born with esotropia, or develop it by 12 months of age, and it is not associated with hyperopia or a high AC/A ratio. In the case of albino children, the cause has been discovered but in the majority of cases it has not. Albino children tend to be esotropic, because of misrouting of fibers in the optic chiasm (Kinnear et al., 1985). The projection from the contralateral eye to the central nervous system is larger than normal (Fig. 6.2), and the projection from the ipsilateral eye is smaller than normal (Creel et al., 1974), as first described in Siamese cats (Guillery, 1969). As a result, there are very few cells with binocular input in the visual cortex, and presumably therefore there is poor control of binocular fusion.

Might other esotropes have a misrouting of fibers at the optic chiasm? In most cases, evidence from evoked potentials in the visual cortex suggests that the projection to the central nervous system is normal (McCormack, 1975; Hoyt and Caltrider, 1984). An exception to this is a class of infantile esotropes with a large angle of deviation, and jerky movements of the eyes (nystagmus). Asymmetric VEPs are seen in these children, although the asymmetry does not always show an enlarged contralateral projection (Ciancia, 1994). In other

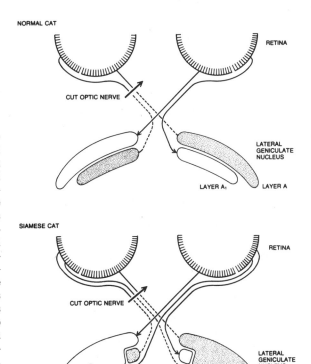

FIG. 6.2. Misrouting of connections in Siamese cats. In normal cats, the nasal half of the retina crosses to the contralateral lateral geniculate nucleus, and the temporal half of the retina projects to the ipsilateral lateral geniculate nucleus (top). In Siamese cats, and other albino animals, some of the temporal half of the retina projects abnormally to the contralateral lateral geniculate (bottom). Consequently, the dividing line between projections that go to one side of the brain as opposed to the other is displaced to the temporal side of the fovea. From Guillery, R. W., 1974, Visual pathways in albinos. Copyright 1974, Scientific American, Inc. All rights reserved.

cases, there could be a misrouting of fibers that does not show up with the VEP techniques that have been used. Regarding this possibility, it is intriguing that strabismus has a genetic component, and that the incidence is higher in light-skinned Caucasians than in dark-skinned non-Caucasians (see Simons, 1993). It is unfortunate that only VEPs have so far been used to study this question, because the technique only reveals gross abnormalities. There is currently no anatomical study of the projections from the eye to the central nervous system in infantile esotropes. Consequently, the question remains unsettled.

There are various hypotheses about the causes of esotropia in unexplained cases. One is that there may be a tendency to develop esotropia because stereopsis for crossed disparity develops before stereopsis for uncrossed disparity (Held, 1993). Crossed disparity is a cue to look at near objects, so this could lead to a tendency toward convergence between the times when crossed and uncrossed disparity develop. However, no study has compared the timing of onset of disparity for crossed compared to uncrossed stimuli in children who become esotropic, to see if this is a tendency that is stronger in such children than in normal children.

Another hypothesis involves the system for detection of movement. There is an interesting correlation in children with infantile esotropia between the development of the esotropia, and the development of monocular optokinetic nystagmus (MOKN). Optokinetic nystagmus can be elicited by allowing a subject to view a drum that has vertical stripes on it, and moves in one direction (Fig. 6.3). The eyes involuntarily follow the drum, then flick back in the reverse direction with a saccade-like eye movement, and the whole cycle is repeated indefinitely. When one eye is open, adults follow the drum equally well in both directions. Normal infants follow the drum better when it is moving in the nasal direction (Atkinson, 1979; Naegele and Held, 1982; see Fig. 6.4). The discrepancy between following in the nasal direction and following in the temporal direction continues until some time between 3 and 6 months.

Adults who had infantile esotropia show the same movement asymmetry that is seen in infants (Atkinson and Braddick, 1981). This is particularly true

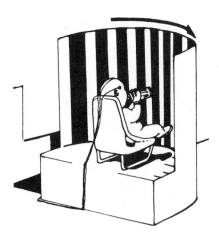

FIG. 6.3. Apparatus used to test optokinetic nystagmus in infants. Infant faces a semicircular screen on which stripes are projected, continually moving in one direction. Reprinted with kind permission from Naegele, J. R., and Held, R., 1982, The postnatal development of monocular optokinetic nystagmus in infants, *Vision Res.* **22**:341–346. Copyright 1982, Elsevier Science, Ltd., The Boulevard, Langford Lane, Kidlington OX5 1GB, UK.

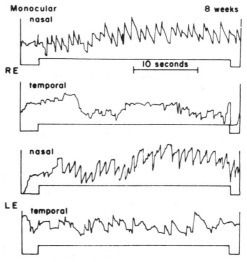

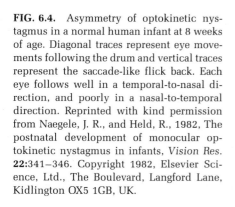

FIG. 6.4. Asymmetry of optokinetic nystagmus in a normal human infant at 8 weeks of age. Diagonal traces represent eye movements following the drum and vertical traces represent the saccade-like flick back. Each eye follows well in a temporal-to-nasal direction, and poorly in a nasal-to-temporal direction. Reprinted with kind permission from Naegele, J. R., and Held, R., 1982, The postnatal development of monocular optokinetic nystagmus in infants, *Vision Res.* **22**:341–346. Copyright 1982, Elsevier Science, Ltd., The Boulevard, Langford Lane, Kidlington OX5 1GB, UK.

when the esotropia appears between birth and 6 months. It happens less frequently when the age of onset is 6–12 months, and is comparatively rare for onset after 1 year of age (Demer and von Noorden, 1988). In addition to an asymmetry in MOKN, there is an asymmetry in judgment of target velocity, and initiation of smooth pursuit eye movements (Tychsen and Lisberger, 1986). Whether the eye movement abnormality leads to esotropia, or esotropia leads to the eye movement abnormality is not known. However, the direction of the asymmetry in the eye movement abnormality is related to the direction of strabismus that is common in infants: movement toward the nose is perceived better, and leads to a stronger eye movement response, and the tendency is for the eyes to turn inward toward the nose (Tychsen and Lisberger, 1986).

Very likely the preference for movements toward the nose is overcome as binocularity and fusion develop (Wattam-Bell *et al.*, 1987). This fits in with the time course of development of various visual properties. Preference for movement toward the nose is present at birth, along with some binocular fixation. During the first 4 months, it gradually disappears. Then, at 4–6 months of age, there is a sudden onset of stereopsis and strong vergence movements. However, more detailed experiments are needed to dissect the cause from the effect.

Sometimes the eyes move together in strabismus, and there is a constant angle of divergence between them (comitant strabismus). Sometimes one eye moves and the other tends not to move (incomitant strabismus). Different strategies are employed in different cases to avoid double vision (diplopia). With incomitant strabismus, the eye that does not move becomes amblyopic and the image in that eye is usually suppressed. With comitant strabismus, the result depends on the angle of deviation (Pasino and Maraini, 1964; see Fig. 6.5). For small angles of deviation, one eye will become amblyopic and this may be enough to avoid double vision (diplopia). For large angles of deviation, suppression may be the main mechanism. For moderate angles of deviation, where the deviation is constant over a substantial period of time, the deviating eye can acquire a new point of fixation which is correlated at some level in the cortex

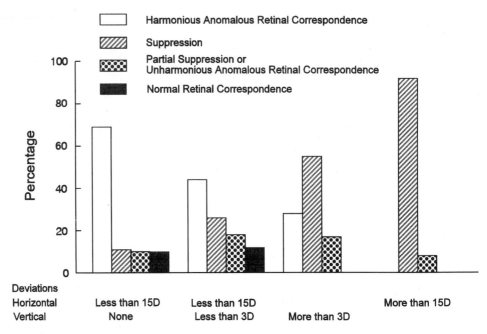

FIG. 6.5. Occurrence of suppression and anomalous retinal correspondence for various degrees of deviation. Reprinted with permission from Pasino, L., and Maraini, G., 1964, *Br. J. Ophthalmol.* **48**:30–34. (Published by BMJ Publishing Group.)

with the projection from the fovea of the normal eye. This is called anomalous retinal correspondence. Strabismic patients who do not suppress the image in one eye will report an extra letter on the Snellen chart (Pugh, 1962; see Fig. 6.6).

Anomalous retinal correspondence can lead to double vision in one eye, if the original projection from the new fixation point in the deviating eye is not eliminated or suppressed. There will be projections from the new fixation point to some portion of the cortex that deals with central vision, and also projections from the new fixation point to the part of the cortex that deals with an area outside central vision, which are the projections that are present at birth. However, this is quite rare.

Exotropia is less common, and even less well understood than esotropia, except in cases with an obvious cause, such as paralysis of the muscle that pulls the eye outward. The general rule is that congenital esotropia is found most frequently before 2 years of age, with an angle of deviation that is large and constant; accommodative esotropia is found most frequently after 2 years of age, with an angle of deviation that is smaller and more variable; and exotropia is found frequently at older ages, and is expressed in an intermittent fashion.

In summary, there are many different types of strabismus and a large number of factors can contribute to them. Development of binocular fusion requires the appropriate quantitative relationship between sensory signals and vergence movements. As discussed in Chapter 3, there is a feedback relationship between increased binocularity and better vergence movements during development. Disruption of the pathway at any point can lead to a lack of binocular

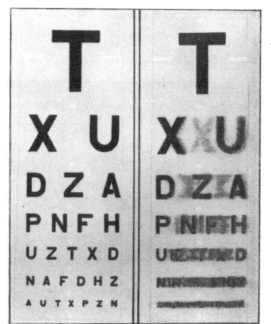

FIG. 6.6. Double vision in a strabismic patient. When asked what she saw on the Snellen chart, an extra X was described on the line of large letters, and the line of small letters was blurred. Reprinted with permission from Pugh, M., 1962, *Br. J. Ophthalmol.* **46**:193–211. (Published by BMJ Publishing Group.)

fusion, and to strabismus. Some contributing factors are understood (a short eyeball, excessive convergence, misrouting of fibers at the optic chiasm) and some are speculative (a tendency to prefer movement toward the nose, a development of crossed stereopsis before uncrossed stereopsis). In a large percentage of cases, exactly what has disturbed the development of binocular fusion and vergence movements is not precisely known.

II. Anisometropia

Anisometropia is a difference in focal point between the two eyes, probably because of a difference in size of the eyeballs. It can lead to amblyopia if the difference persists until the age of 3 years or more (Abrahamsson *et al.*, 1990; von Noordent, 1990). It is associated with strabismus in approximately one-third of the cases. Cause and effect in this association is not clear, because few patients have been followed over a substantial period of time before their amblyopia becomes apparent. In some cases, anisometropia occurs with a very small amount of strabismus (Helveston and von Noorden, 1967). It seems likely in these cases that the anisometropia leads to a poorly defined fixation area in the unfocused eye, which in turn leads to a small angular deviation in the unfocused eye, but it could be the other way around. In other cases, anisometropia develops in the deviating eye after strabismus occurs (Lepard, 1975; see Fig. 6.7). What is known is that acuity in children with both strabismus and anisometropia is worse than acuity in children with strabismus alone, or anisometropia alone (Flom and Bedell, 1985).

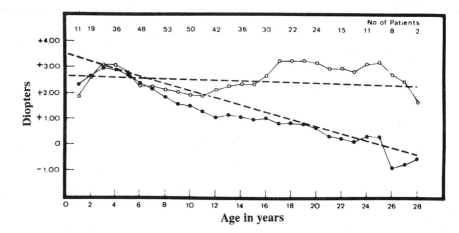

FIG. 6.7. Average refractive error of fixing eyes (closed circles) and amblyopic eyes (open circles) of 55 patients with growth and development at yearly intervals. The amblyopic eye remains hyperopic. The numbers at the top show the number of patients seen at any one age. Reprinted with permission from Lepard, C. W., 1975, *Am. J. Ophthalmol.* **80**:485–490. Copyright by The Ophthalmic Publishing Company.

III. Astigmatism

Astigmatism is a cylindrical component in the refractive system of the eye, usually in the cornea, so that when lines along one axis are in focus, lines along the perpendicular axis are out of focus (Fig. 6.8). A large number of infants have astigmatism at birth, which goes away over the first year of life (Atkinson *et al.*, 1980; see Fig. 6.9). Those who still have significant astigmatism at 1 year of age do not show deficits when the optics of their eyes are corrected (Gwiazda *et al.*, 1985). If the astigmatism persists, however, acuity for lines along the axis of astigmatism becomes poor compared to acuity along the axis in focus, even after correction of the optics, although the evidence for this comes from retrospective studies, and is therefore not unequivocal (Mitchell *et al.*, 1973; see Fig. 6.10).

IV. Cataract

Cataract is a clouding of the lens of the eye. Congenital cataract can be inherited or result from disease such as German measles in the mother. If it is confined to the center of the lens, then light passing through the edge of the lens can form a clear image on the retina. If it covers the whole lens, then the image on the retina is diffused and blurred. The cure is to remove the lens. After this is done, focus of the eye can be corrected for one distance by a spectacle, an intraocular lens implant, or a contact lens, but the eye cannot accommodate. Thus, in cases of unilateral cataract, there will be some anisometropia at some distances. Moreover, depending on the type of optical correction, there will be some difference in the size of the image on the retina between the normal and

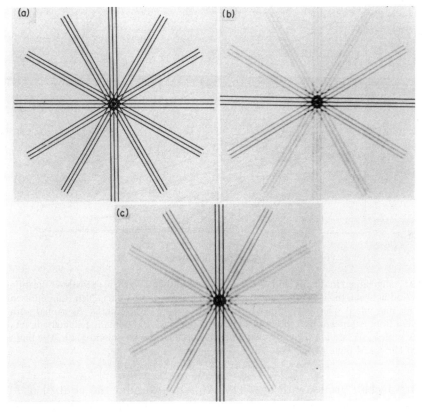

FIG. 6.8. Photographs showing the effect of astigmatic optics on the appearance of objects: (a) as seen by a normal eye; (b) as seen by an eye with astigmatism along the vertical axis; (c) as seen by an eye with astigmatism along the horizontal axis. Reprinted with kind permission from Mitchell, D. E., Freeman, R. D., Millodot, M., and Haegerstrom, G., 1973, Meridional amblyopia: Evidence for modification of the human visual system by early visual experience, *Vision Res.* **13**:535–558. Copyright 1973, Elsevier Science, Ltd., The Boulevard, Langford Lane, Kidlington OX5 1GB, UK.

treated eye. Consequently, the neural changes that can occur after removal of a cataract are extremely hard to treat. Only the most persistent physicians, in collaboration with the most persistent parents, have been successful in treating children with cataracts (Jacobson *et al.*, 1981; Birch *et al.*, 1986; Drummond *et al.*, 1989; Maurer and Lewis, 1993).

V. Myopia

Myopia occurs when the eyeball is too long. If the eyeball is too short, it is farsighted, but one can overcome this to a certain extent by an effort of accommodation. However, one cannot relax the lens much beyond the resting level, and therefore one cannot compensate for an eyeball that is too long. Thus, infants tend to be born hyperopic so that their eyeballs can achieve the correct size by growing (see Fig. 6.7).

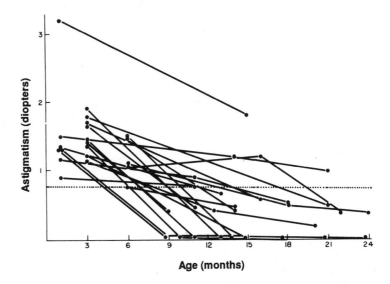

FIG. 6.9. Astigmatism in infants, and its disappearance with age. Vertical axis shows the difference in refraction between the axis of astigmatism and the perpendicular axis. Each line represents the results for one infant who was followed over a period of several months. Reprinted with kind permission from Atkinson, H. J., Braddick, O., and French, J., 1980, Infant astigmatism: Its disappearance with age, *Vision Res.* **20**:891–893. Copyright 1980, Elsevier Science, Ltd., The Boulevard, Langford Lane, Kidlington OX5 1GB, UK.

The eyeball grows with age. This growth is under the control of visual input (see Chapter 13). Over the first few years of life, the growth of the eyeball brings the image into focus on the retina in a relaxed state of accommodation for most people. However, the eyeball cannot shrink. Someone who is born with an eyeball that is too long may be able to compensate for it by a slow rate of

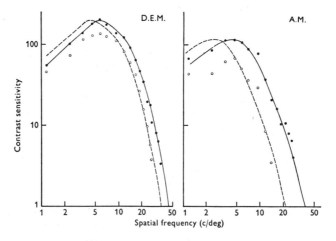

FIG. 6.10. Measurements of contrast sensitivity along the axis of normal focus, and the axis of astigmatism, with corrected optics, for two meridional amblyopes. Acuity, represented by the point where the curve intersects the horizontal axis, was reduced by a factor of 1.5 in D.E.M., and by a factor of 2 in A.M. Reprinted with permission from Mitchell and Wilkinson (1974).

growth, but someone whose eyeball grows to a size that is longer than adult over the first few years of life cannot reverse the process. Thus, the percentage of the population that is myopic increases with age (Curtin, 1985).

Myopia can be brought on by near work, that is, continuous viewing of objects nearby. This point was noted by Kepler in 1611, emphasized by Tscherning in 1882, and has been consistently confirmed since (see Curtin, 1985; Owens, 1991). Interestingly, the prevalence of myopia increases with education: the percentage of myopes goes up from elementary school to middle school to high school, and is highest among university students (Curtin, 1985). Perhaps myopic students tend to become readers rather than football players, but the influence of visual input on the size of the eyeball, to be discussed in Chapter 13, suggests that the reverse is also a definite factor—lots of reading can lead to myopia.

Uncorrected myopia, for strong myopes, leads to a substantial reduction in contrast sensitivity at all spatial frequencies (Fiorentini and Maffei, 1976; see Fig. 6.11). Acuity is reduced, and so is sensitivity to contrast for coarser spatial frequencies. The result of myopia is like that of severe anisometropia, which is to be expected, because they are the same condition, except that the problem occurs in both eyes in the myopia discussed in this section, whereas the problem occurs in one eye in anisometropia, and some anisometropes are hyperopic in their poor eye rather than myopic.

VI. Summary

This short summary shows that a number of different problems can lead to disruption of the signals reaching the visual cortex. On the sensory side there is diffusion of the image on the retina (cataract); poor focus of the image on one retina compared to the other (anisometropia); poor focus along one axis (astig-

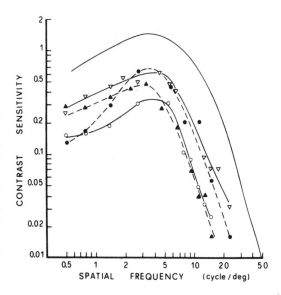

FIG. 6.11. Contrast sensitivity curves from four myopes compared with the normal curve. Top curve shows the contrast sensitivity curve for normal adults. Points and curves drawn through them show the results for the four myopes. Contrast sensitivity is degraded for the myopes at all spatial frequencies. Reprinted with kind permission from Fiorentini, A., and Maffei, L., 1976, Spatial contrast sensitivity of myopic subjects, *Vision Res.* **16**:437–438. Copyright 1976, Elsevier Science, Ltd., The Boulevard, Langford Lane, Kidlington OX5 1GB, UK.

matism); and excessive growth of the eyeball (myopia). On the motor side there are a number of causes of misalignment of the two eyes and mismatch of the information from the two retinas (strabismus). As emphasized in the chapter on development of the visual system, there is an interaction between sensory and motor systems, so that deficits in one will lead to deficits in the other. In all cases there is a danger that the connections in the visual cortex will become rewired to compensate for the deficit, and that the rewiring will become permanent if the underlying deficit is not treated.

References

Abrahamsson, M., Fabian, G., and Sjostrand, J., 1990, A longitudinal study of a population based sample of astigmatic children. II. The changeability of anisometropia, *Acta Ophthalmol.* **68**:435–440.

Atkinson, J., 1979, Development of optokinetic nystagmus in the human infant and monkey infant, in: *Developmental Neurobiology of Vision* (R. D. Freeman, ed.), Plenum Press, New York, pp. 277–287.

Atkinson, J., 1993, Infant vision screening: Prediction and prevention of strabismus and amblyopia from refractive screening in the Cambridge photorefraction program, in: *Early Visual Development, Normal and Abnormal* (K. Simons, ed.), Oxford University Press, London, pp. 335–348.

Atkinson, J., and Braddick, O., 1981, Development of optokinetic nystagmus in the human infant and monkey infant, in: *Eye Movements: Cognition and Perception* (D. F. Fisher, R. A. Monty, and J. W. Senders, eds.), Erlbaum, Hillside, NJ, pp. 53–64.

Atkinson, J., Braddick, O., and French, J., 1980, Infant astigmatism: Its disappearance with age, *Vision Res.* **20**:891–893.

Birch, E. E., Stager, D. R., and Wright, W. W., 1986, Grating acuity development after early surgery for congenital unilateral cataract, *Arch. Ophthalmol.* **104**:1783–1787.

Ciancia, A. O., 1994, On infantile esotropia with nystagmus in abduction, *Trans. ISA Congr.* **7**:1–16.

Creel, D., Witkop, C. J., and King, R. A., 1974, Asymmetric visually evoked potentials in human albinos: Evidence for visual system anomalies, *Invest. Ophthalmol.* **13**:430–440.

Curtin, B. J., 1985, *The Myopias: Basic Science and Clinical Management*, Harper & Row, Philadelphia.

Demer, J. L., and von Noorden, G. K., 1988, Optokinetic asymmetry in esotropia, *J. Pediatr. Ophthalmol. Strabismus* **25**:286–292.

Drummond, G. T., Scott, W. E., and Keach, R. V., 1989, Management of monocular congenital cataracts, *Arch. Ophthalmol.* **107**:45–51.

Fiorentini, A., and Maffei, L., 1976, Spatial contrast sensitivity of myopic subjects, *Vision Res.* **16**:437–438.

Flom, M. C., and Bedell, H. E., 1985, Identifying amblyopia using associated conditions, acuity, and nonacuity features, *Am. J. Optom. Physiol. Opt.* **62**:153–160.

Guillery, R. W., 1969, An abnormal retinogeniculate projection in Siamese cats, *Brain Res.* **14**:739–741.

Guillery, R. W., 1974, Visual pathways in albinos, *Sci. Am.* **230**(5):44–54.

Gwiazda, J., Mohindra, I., Brill, S., and Held, R., 1985, Infant astigmatism and meridional amblyopia, *Vision Res.* **25**:1269–1276.

Held, R., 1993, Two stages in the development of binocular vision and eye alignment, in: *Early Visual Development, Normal and Abnormal* (K. Simons, ed.), Oxford University Press, London, pp. 250–257.

Helveston, E. M., and von Noorden, G. K., 1967, Microtropia, *Arch. Ophthalmol.* **78**:272–281.

Hoyt, C. S., and Caltrider, N., 1984, Hemispheric visually-evoked responses in congenital esotropia, *J. Pediatr. Ophthalmol. Strabismus* **21**:19–21.

Ingram, R. M., Walker, C., Wilson, J. M., Arnold, P. E., and Dally, S., 1986, Prediction of amblyopia and squint by means of refraction at age 1 year, *Br. J. Ophthalmol.* **70**:12–15.

Jacobson, S. G., Mohindra, I., and Held, R., 1981, Development of visual acuity in infants with congenital cataracts, *Br. J. Ophthalmol.* **65:**727–735.

Kinnear, P. E., Jay, B., and Witkop, C. J., 1985, Albinism, *Surv. Ophthalmol.***30:**75–101.

Lepard, C. W., 1975, Comparative changes in the error of refraction between fixing and amblyopic eyes during growth and development, *Am. J. Ophthalmol.* **80:**485–490.

McCormack, E. L., 1975, Electrophysiological evidence for normal optic nerve projections in normally pigmented squinters, *Invest. Ophthalmol.* **14:**931–935.

Maurer, D., and Lewis, T. L., 1993, Visual outcomes after infantile cataract, in: *Early Visual Development, Normal and Abnormal* (K. Simons, ed.), Oxford University Press, London, pp. 454–484.

Mitchell, D. E., and Wilkinson, F. E., 1974, The effect of early astigmatism on the visual resolution of gratings, *J. Physiol. (London)* **243:**739–756.

Mitchell, D. E., Freeman, R. D., Millodot, M., and Haegerstrom, G., 1973, Meridional amblyopia: Evidence for modification of the human visual system by early visual experience, *Vision Res.* **13:**535–558.

Naegele, J. R., and Held, R., 1982, The postnatal development of monocular optokinetic nystagmus in infants, *Vision Res.* **22:**341–346.

Owens, D. A., 1991, Near work, accommodative tonus, and myopia, in: *Refractive Anomalies* (T. Grosvenor and M. C. Flom, eds.), Butterworth–Heinemann, Stoneham, MA, pp. 318–344.

Pasino, L., and Maraini, G., 1964, Importance of natural test conditions in assessing the sensory state of the squinting subject with some clinical considerations on anomalous retinal correspondence, *Br. J. Ophthalmol.* **48:**30–34.

Pugh, M., 1962, Amblyopia and the retina, *Br. J. Ophthalmol.* **46:**193–211.

Simons, K., 1993, Stereoscopic neurontropy and the origins of amblyopia and strabismus, in: *Early Visual Development, Normal and Abnormal* (K. Simons, ed.), Oxford University Press, London, pp. 409–453.

Tychsen, L., and Lisberger, S. G., 1986, Maldevelopment of visual motion processing in humans who had strabismus with onset in infancy, *J. Neurosci.* **6:**2495–2508.

von Noorden, G. K., 1990, *Binocular Vision and Ocular Motility*, Mosby, St. Louis.

Wattam-Bell, J., Braddick, O. J., Atkinson, J., and Day, J., 1987, Measures of infant binocularity in a group at risk for strabismus, *Clin. Vis. Sci.* **1:**327–336.

7

Physiological and Anatomical Changes That Result from Optical and Motor Deficits

Our understanding of what happens in various forms of visual deprivation has increased enormously over the last 35 years, as a result of experiments with animals. The seminal experiments were done by David Hubel and Torsten Wiesel in the early 1960s. They were awarded the Nobel prize in 1981 for this work (Wiesel, 1982), and for their work on the organization of the visual system in normal animals.

I. Monocular Deprivation

The most thorough analysis of the physiological and anatomical changes that occur has been done with regard to monocular deprivation in cats and monkeys. This corresponds to unilateral cataract, which is a comparatively uncommon form of deficit in humans. However, it gives the simplest and clearest results, and is therefore the most useful in pursuing the fundamental mechanisms. The eyelids of one eye are sutured shut for a period of time, resulting in light perception, but very little patterned image on the retina. The direction of movement of an object can be detected through the closed eyelids (Spear et al., 1978), but the shape and form are difficult to see.

If a cat or monkey is monocularly deprived for a period of 3 months from the time of eye opening, it becomes severely amblyopic in that eye (Wiesel and Hubel, 1963b; Dews and Wiesel, 1970). When one records cells in the visual cortex, after opening both eyes for the experiment, very few cells can be activated by the eye that was sutured (Wiesel and Hubel, 1963b; Hubel et al., 1977; see Fig. 7.1). The animal is essentially blind in this eye, because there is little input left from the sutured eye to the visual cortex.

The retina in the sutured eye is normal (Wiesel and Hubel, 1963b; Sherman and Stone, 1973). The physiological properties of cells in the lateral geniculate body that are driven by the sutured eye are grossly normal (Wiesel and Hubel, 1963a). However, the arbors of X (fine detail) cells in the lateral geniculate

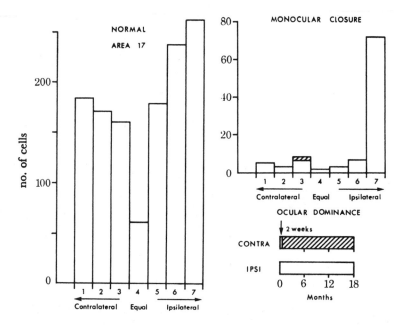

FIG. 7.1. Ocular dominance histograms in normal and monocularly deprived monkeys. A sample of cells is recorded from the visual cortex. Each cell is characterized according to whether it is driven solely by the contralateral eye (group 1), solely by the ipsilateral eye (group 7), equally by both eyes (group 4), or somewhere in between (groups 2, 3, 5, and 6). The histogram on the left was based on 1256 cells recorded from visual cortex in juvenile and adult monkeys. The histogram on the right was obtained from a monkey with the right eye closed from 2 weeks to 18 months, and recordings then made from the left hemisphere. Reprinted with permission from Hubel, D. H., Wiesel, T. N., and LeVay, S., 1977, Plasticity of ocular dominance columns in monkey striate cortex, *Philos. Trans. R. Soc. London Ser. B* **278**:377–409, Fig. 1 (Royal Society, London).

coming from the sutured eye are larger than normal, and the arbors of Y (movement) cells are smaller than normal (Sur *et al.*, 1982). As a result, fewer Y cells are recorded, and the spatial contrast sensitivity of X cells is reduced (see Sherman, 1985).

The major changes that occur are in the projections from the lateral geniculate nucleus to the visual cortex. These can be visualized by putting radioactive amino acids in one eye, which get transported from the eye to the lateral geniculate nucleus and then to the cortex, and mark the input from that eye to layer IV of the cortex. The normal pattern of terminals from one eye is a pattern of stripes, like those on a zebra. When one eye is sutured from an early age, the stripes from the sutured eye are narrower than normal, and the stripes from the open eye are wider (Hubel *et al.*, 1975; see Fig. 7.2). In other words, the terminal arborization in the cortex, coming from cells in the lateral geniculate nucleus driven by the sutured eye, is shrunken (Tieman, 1984). As a result, the cells in the lateral geniculate for this eye are smaller than usual, because they have a smaller terminal arbor to support (Wiesel and Hubel, 1963a).

There are further changes within the cortex. Projections from layer IV to other layers of cortex are also altered to strengthen connections from the open eye, and weaken connections from the sutured eye. This can be deduced from

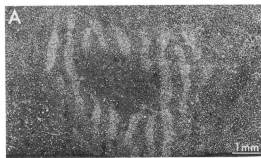

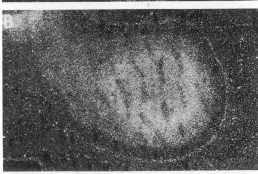

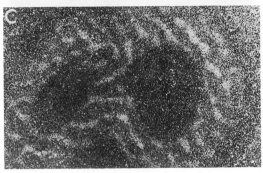

FIG. 7.2. Ocular dominance stripes in layer IV of visual cortex of monkeys. Radioactive tracer is injected into one eye, and transported to the cortex to reveal the projections from that eye. In these sections, cut parallel to the cortical surface, white areas show labelled terminals in layer IV. (A) Normal monkey. (B) Monocularly deprived monkey, normal eye injected, white stripes wider. (C) Monocularly deprived monkey, deprived eye injected, white stripes narrower. Reprinted with permission from Hubel, D. H., Wiesel, T. N., and LeVay, S., 1975, Functional architecture of area 17 in normal and monocularly deprived macaque monkeys, *Cold Spring Harbor Symp. Quant. Biol.* **40:**581–589.

physiological recordings, which show substantial effects in layers II, III, V, and VI when the effects in layer IV are quite small (Shatz and Stryker, 1978; Mower et al., 1985; Daw et al., 1992). It also shows up with anatomical methods that mark the ocular dominance columns in all layers of the cortex (Tumosa et al., 1989).

The effects of monocular deprivation involve competition between the inputs from the two eyes. The effects cannot be explained simply by a loss of connections from the deprived eye. This can be seen by comparing the results from monocular deprivation with those from binocular deprivation. In the case of long-term monocular deprivation from an early age, almost no cells can be driven by the deprived eye. In the case of long-term binocular deprivation, up to one-third of the cells can be driven by one or both eyes and have normal receptive fields (Wiesel and Hubel, 1965). There are a substantial number of cells that do not have visual responses, but the binocular deprivation is not the sum of two monocular deprivations.

To a certain extent, the sculpting of connections that occurs as a result of monocular deprivation is a modification of the changes that occur during development. As described in Chapter 4, the projections from the lateral geniculate nucleus to the visual cortex from the two eyes overlap each other at birth. Then they segregate into eye-specific columns around the time when stereopsis develops. Consequently, the terminals from each eye retract into half the space that they previously occupied. In the case of monocular deprivation, the terminals from the deprived eye retract until they cover a small fraction of the space, and the terminals from the normal eye do not retract. Thus, very few cells in the cortex can be activated by the deprived eye because the input to the cortex from that eye is substantially reduced.

However, the response of the cortex is more complicated than this scenario would suggest. Monocular deprivation continues to have an effect for some time after the process of segregation of afferents from the lateral geniculate to the cortex is finished. Moreover, one can close the left eye until nearly all cells are dominated by the right eye, then open it and close the right eye until nearly all cells are dominated by the left eye, a process known as reverse suture (Blakemore and Van Sluyters, 1974; Movshon, 1976; see Fig. 7.3). Almost certainly, this recovery involves sprouting of terminals, as well as their retraction (LeVay *et al.*, 1980).

Thus, the major effects of monocular deprivation occur within the visual cortex, and involve competition between left and right eye inputs. If the left eye is sutured closed, then there is a retraction of terminals in the visual cortex

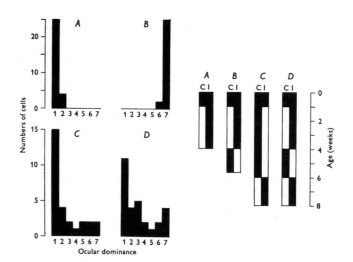

FIG. 7.3. Reversal of the effects of monocular deprivation in cats. Ocular dominance histograms from four animals whose visual experience through the contralateral (C) and ipsilateral (I) eyes is shown on the right. Filled regions indicate periods of eye closure. Closure of the contralateral eye at 4 weeks for 10 days completely reversed the effect of previous closure of the ipsilateral eye (histogram B), and closure at 6 weeks substantially reversed it (histogram C). Reopening the originally open eye at 6 weeks, after 2 weeks of reverse suture, changed the ocular dominance of some cells back again (compare B and D). Reprinted with permission from the Physiological Society, Movshon (1976).

coming from the left eye, and an expansion of terminals coming from the right eye, so that, after a period of time, cells in the visual cortex are driven almost exclusively by the right eye. As a result, in severe cases, the animal becomes almost totally blind in the left eye.

II. Orientation and Direction Deprivation

Changes in the visual cortex also occur from a variety of other forms of visual deprivation. Animals can be reared in an environment of stripes of one orientation. If the stripes are vertical, then there is an increase in the percentage of cells in the visual cortex preferring vertical orientations, and a decrease in the percentage of cells preferring horizontal orientations (Blakemore and Cooper, 1970; Hirsch and Spinelli, 1970; see Fig. 7.4). The opposite occurs for animals reared in an environment of horizontal stripes.

There is an additional change if the stripes are moving in one direction, or if an animal is reared in a pattern of dots moving in one direction. With a stimulus moving to the right, there is an increase in the percentage of cells preferring movement to the right, and a decrease in the percentage of cells preferring movement to the left (Cynader *et al.*, 1975; Daw and Wyatt, 1976; see Fig. 7.5). When the stimulus moves to the left, there is an increase in the percentage of cells preferring movement left.

These effects on orientation and direction selectivity occur in primary visual cortex, which shows the lowest level where such cells are found in higher mammals. There is a rearrangement of the synaptic connections within the visual cortex that produce selectivity for a particular orientation and a

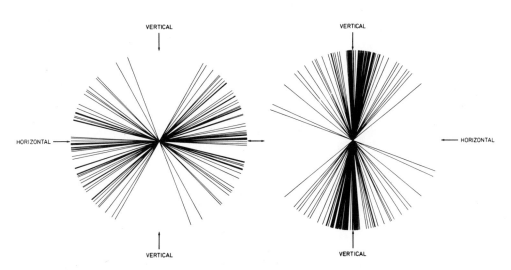

FIG. 7.4. Polar histograms showing the distributions of optimal orientations for 52 neurons from a horizontally experienced cat (left), and 72 neurons from a vertically experienced cat (right). Each line represents the preferred orientation for a single cell in the visual cortex. Reprinted with permission from Blakemore, C., and Cooper, G. F., 1970, Development of the brain depends on the visual environment, *Nature***228**:477–478. Copyright 1970, MacMillan Magazines Limited.

**Normal
Animals**

**Rightward
Reared**

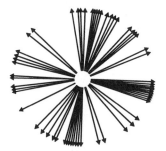
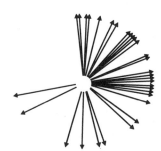

FIG. 7.5. Distribution of preferred directions of direction-selective cells in the cortex of normal animals (left) and the cortex of animals reared in an environment moving to the right (right). Each arrow represents the preferred direction of movement for a single cell. Reprinted with permission from the Physiological Society, Daw and Wyatt (1976).

particular direction. Whether this involves axonal changes, dendritic changes, or just changes in synaptic efficacy is not known, since the synaptic mechanisms underlying orientation and direction selectivity are still controversial, but the effect on the physiological properties of the cells in the cortex is clear.

III. One Eye out of Focus

One eye can be put out of focus by rearing an animal with a substantial concave lens over the eye, sufficiently powerful that the eye cannot accommodate to overcome it. An eye can also be put out of focus by instilling atropine into the conjunctival sac of the eye. This paralyzes accommodation and keeps the pupil dilated. Both methods give the same behavioral result as anisometropia in humans: the contrast sensitivity curve measured through the out-of-focus eye shows reduced contrast sensitivity at medium and high spatial frequencies (Eggers and Blakemore, 1978; Smith *et al.*, 1985; see Fig. 7.6).

The most complete study of the physiological and anatomical results of putting one eye out of focus has been carried out in primates with atropinization of one eye. As with monocular deprivation, the main effect is seen in the visual cortex (Movshon *et al.*, 1987). Cells driven by the atropinized eye have a reduced contrast sensitivity. This effect is most prominent in layers of striate cortex outside layer IV, is noticeable in layer IV, and is not seen in the lateral geniculate nucleus. There is also a reduction in the percentage of binocularly driven neurons, and a small shift in ocular dominance toward the normal eye.

Although physiological techniques do not measure an effect of atropinization on the lateral geniculate, there are anatomical differences (Hendrickson *et al.*, 1987). Cells in layers driven by the atropinized eye are smaller. This is seen in the parvocellular layers, which deal with high spatial frequencies, and not in the magnocellular layers, which deal primarily with movement. As expected, the main effect is found in the pathway that deals with fine details. It is likely

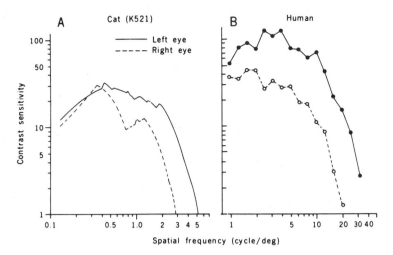

FIG. 7.6. (A) Envelope of contrast sensitivity from cells recorded in the visual cortex of a cat reared with a −12 diopter lens over the right eye. (B) Contrast sensitivity curves for an anisometropic human; normal eye (●), amblyopic eye (○). Reprinted with permission from Eggers, H. M., and Blakemore, C., *Science* **201:**264–266. Copyright 1978, American Association for the Advancement of Science.

that the terminal arbors of these cells are diminished, and that is the cause of the reduction in cell size, so that the anatomical change found in the lateral geniculate is a reflection of changes in the visual cortex.

Thus, results from monocular deprivation and atropinization of one eye are very similar in the level at which they occur. The major physiological effects, which lead to the behavioral consequences of the deficit, occur in primary visual cortex where signals from the two eyes come together.

IV. Strabismus

There are several different ways of creating experimental strabismus. Part of an eye muscle can be removed (myectomy); a tendon cut (tenotomy); an eye muscle cut and reinserted at a different position (recession); botulinum toxin infused into one eye muscle to paralyze it; or base-in prisms placed over the eyes. Strabismus also occurs naturally in a population of cats (Distler and Hoffmann, 1991) and a population of monkeys (Kiorpes and Boothe, 1981), providing useful models for human strabismus. As with humans, these different causes of strabismus have different results. For example, myectomy, tenotomy, or botulinum toxin will produce a pattern of binocular correspondence that varies as the unaffected eye moves (incomitant strabismus), whereas recession or placing prisms over the eyes will produce a binocular mismatch with an angle of mismatch that remains comparatively constant as the eyes move (comitant strabismus).

There are four possible results of strabismus: amblyopia, suppression of the image in one eye, loss of binocular function, and anomalous retinal correspondence. These occur in various combinations in different cases. Loss of

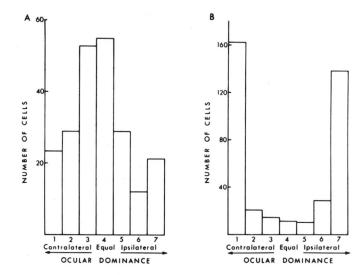

FIG. 7.7. Ocular dominance of 223 cells recorded from normal cats (A) compared to ocular dominance of 384 cells from strabismic cats (B). Reprinted with permission from the *Journal of Neurophysiology*, Hubel and Wiesel (1965).

binocular function is related to a reduction in the number of cells in the visual cortex that can be activated by both eyes. This was first observed by Hubel and Wiesel in cats (1965; see Fig. 7.7), and has been confirmed in all subsequent studies, using a variety of treatments. Along with loss of binocularity goes loss of stereoscopic depth perception (Crawford *et al.*, 1984; Distler and Hoffmann, 1991). The few binocular cells that can be found tend to exhibit a preference for horizontal orientations (Singer *et al.*, 1979; Cynader *et al.*, 1984; see Fig. 7.8). This occurs because the displacement that is created is usually in the horizontal direction. Consequently, a horizontal line may fall within the receptive field of a single cell in the visual cortex, before rewiring takes place, whereas a vertical line probably will not.

Various physiological properties that underlie amblyopia have been found. A reduction in acuity and contrast sensitivity is found in animals with naturally occurring esotropia (Kiorpes and Boothe, 1981), and in various forms of experimental esotropia (von Noorden *et al.*, 1970; von Grunau and Singer, 1980). There may also be a reduction in the number of cells in the visual cortex

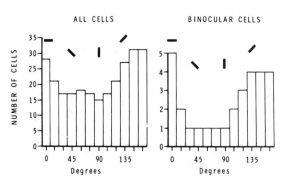

FIG. 7.8. Distribution of preferred orientations among neurons in the visual cortex of strabismic cats. 0° represents cells preferring horizontal orientations, and 90° represents cells preferring vertical. Reprinted with permission from Cynader, M. S., Gardner, J. P., and Mustari, M. J., 1984, Effects of neonatally induced strabismus on binocular responses in cat area 18, *Exp. Brain Res.* **53:**384–399. Copyright 1984, Springer-Verlag.

that are driven by the deviating eye, which is dependent on the part of the field of view that is being recorded (Kalil *et al.*, 1984). Both of these factors contribute to the amblyopia found in esotropic strabismus.

The level at which the reduction in acuity and contrast sensitivity occurs depends on the type of experimental strabismus employed. With tenotomy, there is a small reduction in acuity at the retina/lateral geniculate synapse in cats (Chino *et al.*, 1994), but little is found in primates, and the main part of the deficit occurs in the visual cortex (Crewther and Crewther, 1990). With myectomy, there is a deficit in acuity in the lateral geniculate nucleus (Ikeda and Wright, 1976), which is much more substantial than that found after tenotomy (Crewther *et al.*, 1985). Both procedures produce the same effect as far as the mismatch between the image on the right retina and the image on the left retina is concerned. The difference presumably occurs because removal of part of the body of the eye muscle has some additional effect, perhaps from removal of the input from the sensory endings in the eye muscle, or interference with the blood vessels that penetrate the sclera near the muscle insertion.

Anomalous retinal correspondence is found only when the angle of strabismus is constant and moderate. Presumably, axons in the cortex can find their way to a new location that is nearby, but not to a new location that is a long distance away. In experiments on cats, anomalous retinal correspondence is seen with angles of strabismus less than 10° (Grant and Berman, 1991; see Fig. 7.9).

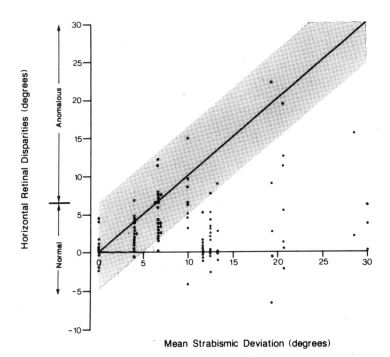

FIG. 7.9. Retinal correspondence found in binocular cells from area LS in cats with various degrees of strabismus. For cells with normal or innate correspondence, the disparity will be 0°. For cells with anomalous correspondence that will produce a single image, the disparity will equal the degree of strabismic deviation (45° line). Cells with anomalous correspondence are not seen very often when the strabismic deviation is greater than 10°. From Grant and Berman *Vis. Neurosci.* 7:259–281 (1991). Reprinted with the permission of Cambridge University Press.

Cortical cells with anomalous retinal correspondence are not found in primary visual cortex (area 17). They are found in the lateral suprasylvian gyrus of the cat (LS), which contains several areas of secondary visual cortex (Grant and Berman, 1991; Sireteanu and Best, 1992), and some are also found in area 18 (Cynader *et al.*, 1984). Cells in primary visual cortex tend to have small receptive fields, while cells in LS tend to have large ones. Thus, in the normal animal, a point in LS will receive input from a wide area of retina, and the axon terminals will not have to move a long distance in order to get anomalous retinal correspondence. Essentially what happens with small angles of strabismus is that the cells in primary visual cortex become monocular, and the site of binocular convergence is moved to secondary visual cortex, where the compensation for the lack of correspondence in the retina takes place.

Where the images in the two eyes cannot be brought together through anomalous retinal correspondence, because the distance that the axon terminals in the cortex would have to move is too large, there will be two images reaching the visual cortex that are not in register. In this case, one image is inhibited or suppressed. The mechanism of image suppression is still not fully understood. Inhibition of the cortical response from the deviated eye by stimulation of the nondeviated eye has been seen (Singer *et al.*, 1980; Freeman and Tsumoto, 1983; Crewther and Crewther, 1993). Freeman and Tsumoto (1983) reported that the frequency and strength of the inhibition in exotropic cats was similar to that seen in normal cats, while the deviated eye was more effectively suppressed by and less able to suppress the nondeviated eye in esotropic cats (Fig. 7.10). This tallies with the clinical observation that there is a tendency for exotropes to have alternating fixation, while esotropes tend to fixate with their normal eye, and become amblyopic in the deviating eye. Suppression seen in strabismic cats may be similar to interocular suppression seen in normal cats, except that it occurs with stimuli of the same orientation, as well as with stimuli of different orientation (Sengpiel *et al.*, 1994). However, the precise mechanism of inhibition, whether it varies from one part of the field of view to another, and how it varies in esotropia with the angle of strabismus all remain to be investigated.

V. Summary

The general conclusion is that mammals compensate for optical deficits occurring at a young age by anatomical and physiological changes in the visual cortex. Not much compensation is found at the level of the retina or the lateral geniculate nucleus. In the case of binocular function, orientation selectivity, and direction selectivity, this is what one would expect, because these are all properties of the visual cortex rather than the retina or lateral geniculate. The mechanisms that produce acuity and contrast sensitivity changes are also often found at the cortical level, even though acuity and contrast sensitivity are basically properties of the retina and lateral geniculate.

The compensation is specific for the deficit. Monocular deprivation affects ocular dominance rather than orientation selectivity, and orientation deprivation affects orientation selectivity rather than ocular dominance. There is a

ESO

NON-DEV.   **DEV.**

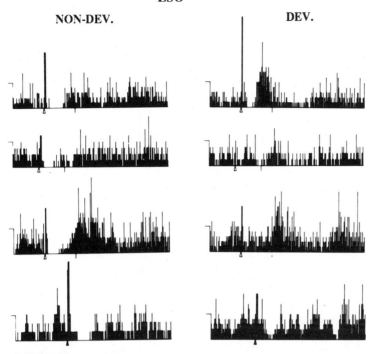

FIG. 7.10. Inhibition is seen when the nondeviating eye is stimulated more than when the deviating eye is stimulated. Records from cells in the visual cortex of an esotropic cat. Reprinted with permission from the *Journal of Neurophysiology*, Freeman and Tsumoto (1983).

rearrangement of the connections within the cortex, and the columns specific for the deprived features contract, while the columns specific for the non-deprived features expand. The physiological properties of the cells change correspondingly.

There is a limit as to how far compensation can occur through anatomical rearrangements. This is not important for monocular, orientation, and direction deprivation, because columns for left and right eyes are near each other, and so are columns for vertical and horizontal orientations, and cells for rightward and leftward movement. It is, however, important for strabismus, when the angle of strabismus is large. In this case, compensation occurs through some form of physiological suppression rather than through anatomical rearrangements.

References

Blakemore, C., and Cooper, G. F., 1970, Development of the brain depends on the visual environment, *Nature* **228**:477–478.

Blakemore, C., and Van Sluyters, R. C., 1974, Reversal of the physiological effects of monocular deprivation in kittens: Further evidence for a sensitive period, *J. Physiol. (London)* **237**:195–216.

Chino, Y. M., Cheng, H., Smith, E. L., Garraghty, P. E., Roe, A. W., and Sur, M., 1994, Early discordant binocular vision disrupts signal transfer in the lateral geniculate nucleus, *Proc. Natl. Acad. Sci. USA* **91**:6938–6942.

Crawford, M. L. J., Smith, E. L., Harwerth, R. S., and von Noorden, G. K., 1984, Stereoblind monkeys have few binocular neurons, *Invest. Ophthalmol. Vis. Sci.* **25**:779–781.

Crewther, D. P., and Crewther, S. G., 1990, Neural site of strabismic amblyopia in cats: Spatial frequency deficit in primary cortical neurons, *Exp. Brain Res.* **79**:615–622.

Crewther, S. G., and Crewther, D. P., 1993, Amblyopia and suppression in binocular cortical neurones of strabismic cat, *Neurosci. Res.* **4**:1083–1086.

Crewther, S. G., Crewther, D. P., and Cleland, B. G., 1985, Convergent strabismic amblyopia in cats, *Exp. Brain Res.* **60**:1–9.

Cynader, M. S., Berman, N., and Hein, A., 1975, Cats raised in a one-directional world: Effects on receptive fields in visual cortex and superior colliculus, *Exp. Brain Res.* **22**:267–280.

Cynader, M. S., Gardner, J. P., and Mustari, M. J., 1984, Effects of neonatally induced strabismus on binocular responses in cat area 18, *Exp. Brain Res.* **53**:384–399.

Daw, N. W., and Wyatt, H. J., 1976, Kittens reared in a unidirectional environment: Evidence for a critical period, *J. Physiol. (London)* **257**:155–170.

Daw, N. W., Fox, K., Sato, H., and Czepita, D., 1992, Critical period for monocular deprivation in the cat visual cortex, *J. Neurophysiol.* **67**:197–202.

Dews, P. D., and Wiesel, T. N., 1970, Consequences of monocular deprivation on visual behaviour in kittens, *J. Physiol. (London)* **206**:437–455.

Distler, C., and Hoffmann, K. P., 1991, Depth perception and cortical physiology in normal and innate microstrabismic cats, *Vis. Neurosci.* **6**:25–41.

Eggers, H. M., and Blakemore, C., 1978, Physiological basis of anisometropic amblyopia, *Science* **201**:264–266.

Freeman, R. D., and Tsumoto, T., 1983, An electrophysiological comparison of convergent and divergent strabismus in the cat: Electrical and visual activation of single cortical cells, *J. Neurophysiol.* **49**:238–253.

Grant, S., and Berman, N. E. J., 1991, Mechanism of anomalous retinal correspondence: Maintenance of binocularity with alteration of receptive-field position in the lateral suprasylvian (LS) visual area of strabismic cats, *Vis. Neurosci.* **7**:259–281.

Hendrickson, A. E., Movshon, J. A., Eggers, H. M., Gizzi, M. S., Boothe, R. G., and Kiorpes, L., 1987, Effects of early unilateral blur on the macaques's visual system. II. Anatomical observations, *J. Neurosci.* **7**:1327–1339.

Hirsch, H. V. B., and Spinelli, D. N., 1970, Visual experience modifies distribution of horizontally and vertically oriented receptive fields in cats, *Science* **168**:869–871.

Hubel, D. H., and Wiesel, T. N., 1965, Binocular interaction in striate cortex of kittens reared with artificial squint, *J. Neurophysiol.* **28**:1041–1059.

Hubel, D. H., Wiesel, T. N., and LeVay, S., 1975, Functional architecture of area 17 in normal and monocularly deprived macaque monkeys, *Cold Spring Harbor Symp. Quant. Biol.* **40**:581–589.

Hubel, D. H., Wiesel, T. N., and LeVay, S., 1977, Plasticity of ocular dominance columns in monkey striate cortex, *Philos. Trans. R. Soc. London Ser. B.* **278**:377–409.

Ikeda, H., and Wright, M. J., 1976, Properties of LGN cells in kittens reared with convergent squint: A neurophysiological demonstration of amblyopia, *Exp. Brain Res.* **25**:63–77.

Kalil, R. E., Spear, P. D., and Langsetmo, A., 1984, Response properties of striate cortex neurons in cats raised with divergent or convergent strabismus, *J. Neurophysiol.* **52**:514–537.

Kiorpes, L., and Boothe, R. G., 1981, Naturally occurring strabismus in monkeys (Macaca nemestrina), *Invest. Ophthalmol. Vis. Sci.* **20**:257–263.

LeVay, S., Wiesel, T. N., and Hubel, D. H., 1980, The development of ocular dominance columns in normal and visually deprived monkeys, *J. Comp. Neurol.* **1991**:1–51.

Movshon, J. A., 1976, Reversal of the physiological effects of monocular deprivation in the kitten's visual cortex, *J. Physiol. (London)* **261**:125–174.

Movshon, J. A., Eggers, H. M., Gizzi, M. S., Hendrickson, A. E., Kiorpes, L., and Boothe, R. G., 1987, Effects of early unilateral blur on the macaque's visual system. III. Physiological observations, *J. Neurosci.* **7**:1340–1351.

Mower, G. D., Caplan, C. J., Christen, W. G., and Duffy, F. H., 1985, Dark rearing prolongs physiological but not anatomical plasticity of the cat visual cortex, *J. Comp. Neurol.* **235:**448–466.

Sengpiel, F., Blakemore, C., Kind, P. C., and Harrad, R., 1994, Interocular suppression in the visual cortex of strabismic cats, *J. Neurosci.* **14:**6855–6871.

Shatz, C. J., and Stryker, M. P., 1978, Ocular dominance in layer IV of the cat's visual cortex and the effects of monocular deprivation, *J. Physiol. (London)* **281:**267–283.

Sherman, S. M., 1985, Development of retinal projections to the cat's lateral geniculate nucleus, *Trends Neurosci.* **8:**350–355.

Sherman, S. M., and Stone, J., 1973, Physiological normality of the retina in visually deprived cats, *Brain Res.* **60:**224–230.

Singer, W., Rauschecker, J., and von Grunau, M., 1979, Squint affects striate cortex cells encoding horizontal image movements, *Brain Res.* **170:**182–186.

Singer, W., von Grunau, M. W., and Rauschecker, J. P., 1980, Functional amblyopia in kittens with unilateral exotropia. I. Electrophysiological assessment, *Exp. Brain Res.* **40:**294–304.

Sireteanu, R., and Best, J., 1992, Squint-induced modification of visual receptive fields in the lateral suprasylvian cortex of the cat: Binocular interaction, vertical effect and anomalous correspondence, *Eur. J. Neurosci.* **4:**235–242.

Smith, E. L., Harwerth, R. S., and Crawford, M. L. J., 1985, Spatial contrast sensitivity deficits in monkeys produced by optically induced anisometropia, *Invest. Ophthalmol. Vis. Sci.* **26:**330–342.

Spear, P. D., Tong, L., and Langsetmo, A., 1978, Striate cortex neurons of binocularly deprived kittens respond to visual stimuli through the closed eyelids, *Brain Res.* **155:**141–146.

Sur, M., Humphrey, A. H., and Sherman, S. M., 1982, Monocular deprivation affects X- and Y-cell terminations in cats, *Nature* **300:**183–185.

Tieman, S. B., 1984, Effects of monocular deprivation on geniculocortical synapses in the cat, *J. Comp. Neurol.* **222:**166–176.

Tumosa, N., Tieman, S. B., and Tieman, D. G., 1989, Binocular competition affects the pattern and intensity of ocular activation columns in the visual cortex of cats, *Vis. Neurosci.* **2:**391–407.

von Grunau, M. W., and Singer, W., 1980, Functional amblyopia in kittens with unilateral exotropia. II. Correspondence between behavioural and electrophysiological assessment, *Exp. Brain Res.* **40:**305–310.

von Noorden, G. K., Dowling, J. E., and Ferguson, D. C., 1970, Experimental amblyopia in monkeys, *Arch. Ophthalmol.* **84:**206–214.

Wiesel, T. N., 1982, Postnatal development of the visual cortex and the influence of environment, *Nature* **299:**583–591.

Wiesel, T. N., and Hubel, D. H., 1963a, Effects of visual deprivation on morphology and physiology of cells in the cat's lateral geniculate body, *J. Neurophysiol.* **26:**978–993.

Wiesel, T. N., and Hubel, D. H., 1963b, Single cell responses in striate cortex of kittens deprived of vision in one eye, *J. Neurophysiol.* **26:**1003–1017.

Wiesel, T. N., and Hubel, D. H., 1965, Comparison of the effects of unilateral and bilateral eye closure on cortical unit responses in kittens, *J. Neurophysiol.* **28:**1029–1040.

8

What Is Amblyopia?

Amblyopia was originally defined as poor vision, or blunt sight. The aspect of the deficit that is most commonly characterized is acuity, usually in the ophthalmologist's office with a Snellen chart. However, the deficit as a whole is much more complicated than this. There may be a loss of connections or a distortion or rearrangement of connections within the visual cortex. What happens varies, according to the problem that caused the deficit, because the compensation in the central nervous system is specific to the optical or motor problem that has to be compensated. In some cases, as we shall see, there can even be a distortion of vision without any loss of acuity. Thus, amblyopia covers a variety of different forms of poor vision. As far as is currently possible, this chapter will describe the variations.

Amblyopia has been studied almost entirely by psychophysical means. However, some of the most interesting observations have come from asking patients what they see. One can make psychophysical measurements, such as contrast sensitivity, in animals, and tally the results with anatomical and physiological measurements. Unfortunately, one cannot ask the animals what they see. Thus, the anatomical and physiological mechanisms that underlie details of the various forms of amblyopia are, in many cases, speculative. One can make some suggestions, based on what is known and has been described in the last chapter. However, experiments that prove the suggestions remain to be done.

I. Amblyopia from Anisometropia

The easiest situation to describe and to understand is anisometropia. In cases where there is no strabismus, the two eyes look in approximately the same direction. Most of the time the image in one eye is out of focus, and therefore the image on the retina is degraded. As a result, the connections between the retina and the cortex do not form as precise a topographic map as they do in a normal person. We do not yet know if the normal topographic map forms and then degenerates, or if there is a process of refinement of the topographic map over the first few years of life that does not occur when the image on the retina is out of focus. In any case, the image is poor and vision is poor over most of the field of view of one eye.

Acuity as measured by gratings is diminished in the amblyopic eye, and so is contrast sensitivity. The contrast sensitivity curve tends to have substantial losses at high spatial frequencies, and not much loss at low spatial frequencies (Bradley and Freeman, 1981). Acuity can be measured with gratings or with letters, and the results correspond with each other (Levi and Klein, 1982). Vernier acuity is also reduced. The fraction by which acuity is reduced varies from patient to patient, but for a particular patient, vernier, grating, and Snellen acuity are all reduced by the same fraction (Levi and Klein, 1982; see Fig. 8.1). The acuity loss is also found in the peripheral part of the field of view, equally in both nasal and temporal parts of the field (Sireteanu and Fronius, 1981). This suggests that the grain of the whole system is degraded by an amount that depends on the extent of the anisometropia.

Interestingly, monocularly driven acuity is spared. In the far periphery of the temporal field, there is a part of the field of view that is driven by one eye only. This is the monocular part of the field of view. In this area, anisometropic

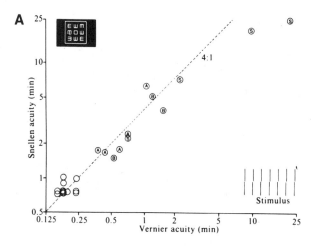

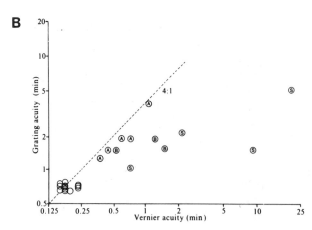

FIG. 8.1. Relationship between (A) Snellen acuity and vernier acuity; and (B) grating acuity and vernier acuity for anisometropic amblyopes Ⓐ, strabismic amblyopes Ⓑ, amblyopes that are both anisometropic and strabismic Ⓢ, and normal people ○. For anisometropic amblyopes, grating acuity, vernier acuity, and letter (Snellen) acuity are linearly related. Reprinted with permission from Levi, D. M., and Klein, S., 1982, Hyperacuity and amblyopia, *Nature* **298:**268–270. Copyright 1982, MacMillan Magazines Limited.

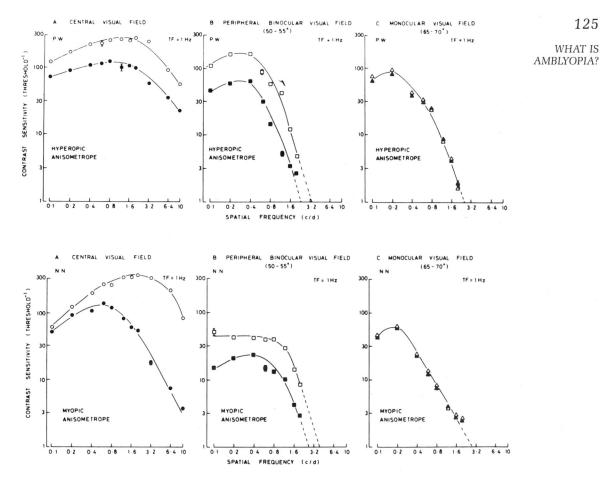

FIG. 8.2. Contrast sensitivity in binocular and monocular parts of the field of view for two hyperopic anisometropes. Filled symbols show contrast sensitivity in amblyopic eye, and open symbols contrast sensitivity in normal eye. Reprinted with kind permission from Hess, R. F., and Pointer, J. S., 1985, Differences in the neural basis of amblyopia: The distribution of the anomaly across the visual field, *Vision Res.* **25**:1577–1594. Copyright 1985, Elsevier Science, Ltd., The Boulevard, Langford Lane, Kidlington OX5 1GB, UK.

amblyopes do not show deficits (Hess and Pointer, 1985; see Fig. 8.2). Consequently, there must be binocular interactions leading to the deficits seen in the binocular part of the field of view. Presumably the good eye competes with the blurred eye, and takes over space in the cortex from the blurred eye, just as it does in monocular deprivation. This tallies with the small shift in ocular dominance found in the animal model.

Spatial localization is degraded in anisometropic amblyopes in proportion to their contrast sensitivity loss (Hess and Holliday, 1992). To test this, one needs a stimulus that is devoid of local vernier cues. Hess and Holliday used a triplet of "Gabor patches" (Fig. 8.3), with the task of lining up the middle one between the upper and lower ones. Anisometropic amblyopes showed no defi-

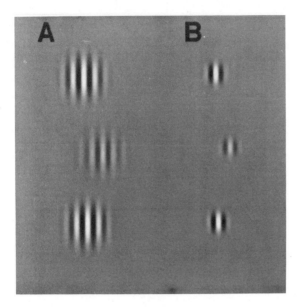

FIG. 8.3. A task used to test spatial uncertainty in amblyopes. The task is to line up the middle "Gabor patch" between the upper and lower ones. Reprinted with kind permission from Hess, R. F., and Holliday, I. E., 1992, The spatial localization deficit in amblyopia, *Vision Res.* **32:**1319–1339. Copyright 1992, Elsevier Science, Ltd., The Boulevard, Langford Lane, Kidlington OX5 1GB, UK.

cit when the elements were set to be the same fraction above threshold for both normal and amblyopic eyes.

In sum, different anisometropes show different losses in acuity and contrast sensitivity, depending on the extent of their anisometropia. However, losses in other parameters that have been measured, such as vernier acuity and spatial localization, are scaled in proportion to their acuity loss. The system acts as though there is a blurring of the connections between retina and cortex, which affects all aspects of visual performance equally.

II. Effect of Cataracts

Amblyopia resulting from cataract is called stimulus-deprivation amblyopia. In untreated cases the effect is much worse than in anisometropia or strabismus. In unilateral cataract the input from the deprived eye to the cortex is virtually lost, whereas in anisometropia this input is reduced a little, and is not as precise as normal. Consequently, many children with congenital untreated unilateral cataract have an acuity of less than 20/200 (1/10th normal) and are legally blind (Maurer and Lewis, 1993; see Fig. 8.4A). The therapy is to remove the cataract surgically, provide optical correction to compensate for the loss of the lens, and then to patch the good eye for 40–50% of the time each day to force the child to use the poor eye. Even this is not totally effective (Fig. 8.4A). Children with congenital bilateral cataract are better off, but their vision is still substantially below normal (Fig. 8.4B).

III. Amblyopia from Strabismus

The deficits caused by strabismus are more complicated. Sometimes the angle of deviation is quite small. In these cases the result is not very different

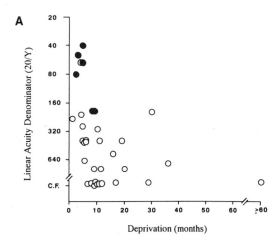

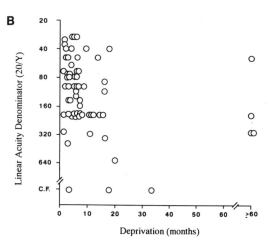

FIG. 8.4. (A) Linear letter acuity for children with unilateral cataract, as a function of the duration of deprivation. In some cases the good eye was patched 40–50% of the waking time (●), and in some cases it was not (○). (B) Linear letter acuity as a function of the duration of deprivation in children treated for bilateral congenital cataracts. From Maurer and Lewis, *Early Visual Development: Normal and Abnormal*, Kurt Simons, ed. Copyright © 1993 by Oxford University Press, Inc. Reprinted by permission.

from that in anisometropia. There will be poor acuity and poor contrast sensitivity in the wandering eye.

Sometimes there is a new point of fixation away from the fovea. This occurs mainly in cases of esotropia, where the angle of deviation is not too large, and remains constant during early development to enable the new fixation point to be established. Connections may form from the new point of fixation to higher areas of cortex dealing with central vision, to create anomalous retinal correspondence, as discussed in previous chapters.

Acuity at the new point of fixation is limited by the density of ganglion cells in the retina, and the size of the center of their receptive fields. The size of the center of the receptive field gets larger, and the density per unit area of retina gets lower, as one moves away from the fovea (Fig. 8.5). This puts a limit on the acuity that can be obtained. No matter how precisely the connections between retina and cortex are rearranged, acuity can never be better than the spacing of ganglion cells in the retina. However, acuity is frequently worse than this limit, showing that there is also a muddling of connections between the new point of fixation and the cortex (Hess, 1977).

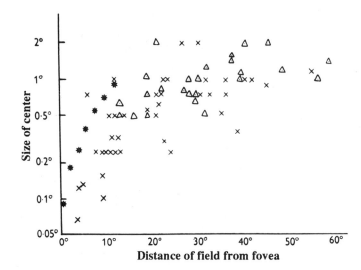

FIG. 8.5. Decrease in spatial summation away from the fovea, related to increase in the size of the center of receptive fields in the retina. X indicate ON-center units, and △ OFF-center cells from Hubel and Wiesel (1960). Asterisks represent minimum of the Westheimer function (a measurement of summation area) in normal human eyes. From Enoch et al. (1970). Reprinted by permission of Kluwer Academic Publishers.

Despite the fact that the visual center has changed, the fovea still exists, with a high density of receptors, ganglion cells, and lateral geniculate cells per unit area of retina. Consequently, vision is clearest away from the point of fixation in the direction of the fovea. This is illustrated in Fig. 8.6 from Pugh (1962). The subject was amblyopic in the left eye with esotropia and some hypotropia. Thus, the fovea was to the left and above the point of fixation, and the direction of clearest vision was to the right and below. The right-hand side of objects was seen more clearly than the left.

As illustrated in Fig. 8.6, the small letters on the Snellen chart tend to run together. The latter is called separation difficulty, or the crowding effect (Irvine, 1948; Stuart and Burian, 1962). As a result, acuity for single letters is better than acuity for letters in a line. Irvine stated that "others describe a crowding together of the letters on a line as if the macular area and a portion of the retina to one side of it project in almost the same direction."

The crowding phenomenon occurs in normal people as well as in amblyopes (Stuart and Burian, 1962; Flom et al., 1963). For any person, the presence of an object affects the visibility of an object nearby. Probably this occurs because the cells in the visual cortex that analyze orientation of edges and form for one location interact with similar cells for a neighboring location. In the case of anisometropic amblyopes, the magnitude of the crowding effect is proportional to the degradation in acuity (Levi and Klein, 1985). In the case of strabismic amblyopes, as expected from the nature of the rearrangement of the connections between retina and cortex, the crowding deficit can be much greater than the acuity deficit (Levi and Klein, 1985).

There is a wide variety of compensating rearrangements of the connections

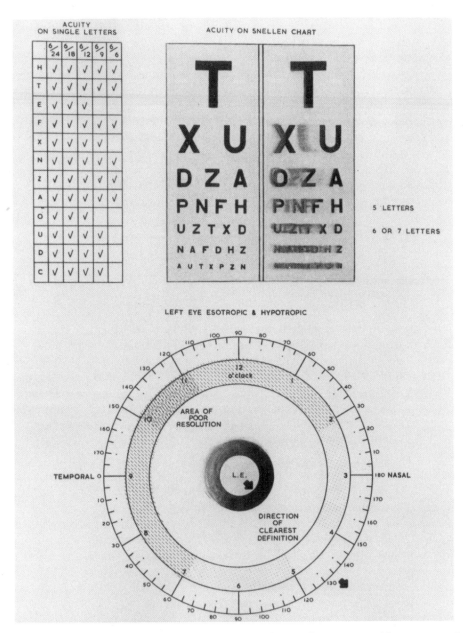

FIG. 8.6. Illustration of what an amblyope sees, for a subject with esotropia and hypotropia in the left eye. Objects were clearer on the right side than on the left. A second letter was seen between the large letters on the Snellen chart. For the smaller letters on the chart, they tended to run together. Consequently, acuity for single letters was better than acuity for letters in a line (crowding phenomenon). Reprinted with permission from Pugh, M. G., 1962, *Br. J. Ophthalmol.* **46**:193–211. (Published by BMJ Publishing Group.)

between retina and cortex. Presumably this is related to the direction and extent of the deviation of the eye during the first few months of life, and whether this deviation is constant or variable. One only discovers this variability by asking the patient what he or she sees—something that, with one or two exceptions, is not reported in the scientific literature. Some of the variations are illustrated neatly by Hess *et al.* (1978), who measured contrast sensitivity curves in a number of patients, and also asked them what the gratings looked like.

Some patients who saw distorted gratings reported normal contrast sensitivity (Fig. 8.7). For others who had normal contrast sensitivity, part of the grating disappeared at fine spatial frequencies (Fig. 8.8). Presumably in these cases enough fine-grain foveal connections were still there to give normal acuity. However, there is some scrambling of connections in areas of central vision, and the nature of these varies from case to case.

In other cases, patients reported degraded contrast sensitivity and a variety of deficits in the detailed perception of the grating. An example is given in Fig. 8.9: in this case, the lines in the grating appeared to be broken up. Obviously the results also depend on the size and position of the test grating. A large grating will cover a large area of retina, and the orientation of the grating can be detected by any part of the field of view that is included. Results with a small grating will depend on where it is placed in the field of view. This point is particularly true when the part of the retina that is amblyopic is large (Fig. 8.10).

The results of Hess *et al.*, help to explain why letter acuity is worse than grating acuity—an observation that has been known for a long time (Gstalder and Green, 1971). This is not just an example of the crowding phenomenon,

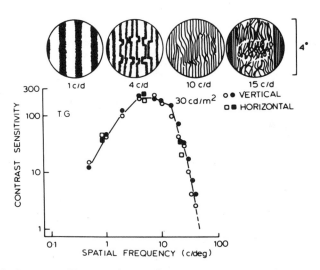

FIG. 8.7. Results from an amblyope with normal contrast sensitivity, and distorted vision. Results from the amblyopic eye shown with filled symbols, and for the normal eye with open symbols. Contrast sensitivity curves at the bottom: what the amblyope saw shown at the top. Reprinted with permission from Hess, R. F., Campbell, F. W., and Greenhalgh, T., 1978, On the nature of the neural abnormality in human amblyopia: Neural aberrations and neural sensitivity loss, *Pfluegers Arch. Gesamte Physiol.* **377:**201–207. Copyright 1978, Springer-Verlag.

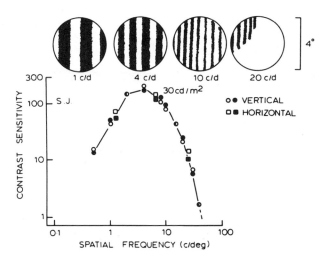

FIG. 8.8. Results from an amblyope with normal contrast sensitivity, but poor acuity in one part of the field of view. Reprinted with permission from Hess, R. F., Campbell, F. W., and Greenhalgh, T., 1978, On the nature of the neural abnormality in human amblyopia: Neural aberrations and neural sensitivity loss, *Pfluegers Arch. Gesamte Physiol.* **377**:201–207. Copyright 1978, Springer-Verlag.

because acuity for single letters is worse than grating acuity, as well as acuity for letters in a line (Katz and Sireteanu, 1990; see Fig. 8.11). Two factors combine to produce this result. One is simply that a grating can be detected if it is visible in any part of the field of view that it covers. The other is that local distortions of the image make the details of letters hard to see.

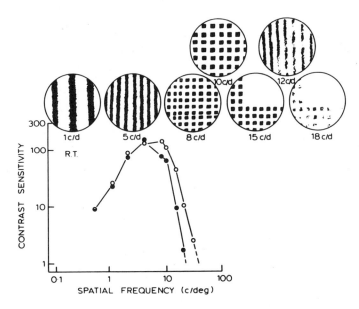

FIG. 8.9. An amblyope with loss of contrast sensitivity, where the lines of the grating appeared broken up. Reprinted with permission from Hess, R. F., Campbell, F. W., and Greenhalgh, T., 1978, On the nature of the neural abnormality in human amblyopia: Neural aberrations and neural sensitivity loss, *Pfluegers Arch. Gesamte Physiol.* **377**:201–207. Copyright 1978, Springer-Verlag.

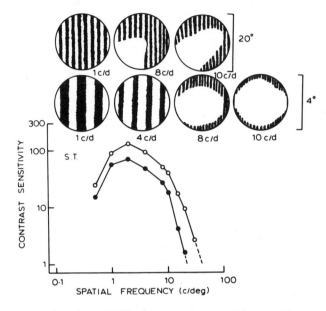

FIG. 8.10. Appearance of gratings of different sizes, for an amblyope with a scotoma in central vision. Reprinted with permission from Hess, R. F., Campbell, F. W., and Greenhalgh, T., 1978, On the nature of the neural abnormality in human amblyopia: Neural aberrations and neural sensitivity loss, *Pfluegers Arch. Gesamte Physiol.* **377**:201–207. Copyright 1978, Springer-Verlag.

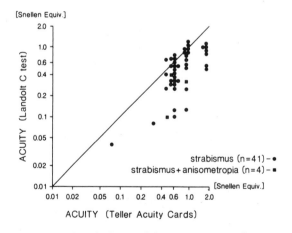

FIG. 8.11. Letter acuity measured with the Landolt C test, compared to grating acuity measured with Teller acuity cards. In the Landolt C test, the task is to detect the gap in a "C," when it is presented in one of four different directions. With Teller acuity cards, the patient is presented with a grating and a uniform card, and an observer states which the patient spends more time looking at. Acuity with the Landolt C test is frequently worse, and never significantly better than with Teller acuity cards. Reprinted with kind permission from Katz, B., and Sireteanu, R. W., 1990, The Teller acuity card test: A useful method for the clinical routine? *Clin. Vision Sci.* **5**:307–323. Copyright 1985, Elsevier Science, Ltd., The Boulevard, Langford Lane, Kidlington OX5 1GB, UK.

The same point can be seen in a study of vernier acuity. One can express vernier acuity as a percentage of the resolution limit, measured with a grating. For normal eyes, this percentage is about 16%. If the vernier acuity is measured with a pair of gratings offset from each other (see Fig. 3.7), there is an increase in this percentage when the gratings are fine, within 1 octave (a factor of 2) of the resolution limit (Levi and Klein, 1982; see Fig. 8.12). Results in anisometropic amblyopes are similar to normal. However, results in strabismic amblyopes are very different: vernier acuity is substantially more than 16% of grating acuity when the spatial frequency of the display is less than 3 octaves below the resolution limit.

This loss of vernier acuity is a form of "spatial uncertainty" at a fine level, in the sense that amblyopes cannot tell where one grating is in relation to the other. Spatial uncertainty at a coarse level is also worse in strabismic amblyopes than in anisometropic amblyopes. This deficit can be seen in a bisection task, where the amblyope is asked to line up a short line with markers above and below it, or place it midway between two others on each side of it (Flom and Bedell, 1985; see Fig. 8.13A). It can also be seen in a placing task, where the amblyope is asked to arrange a sequence of dots so as to be equidistant from a central fixation point. The result can be distinctly asymmetric (Fig. 8.13B), although deficits of this magnitude are fairly rare. While spatial uncertainty in

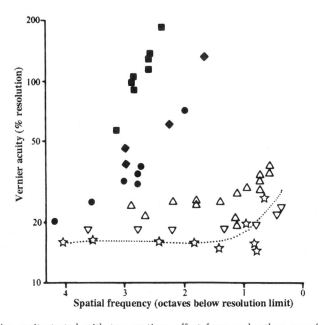

FIG. 8.12. Vernier acuity tested with two gratings offset from each other, as a function of the fundamental frequency of the grating. Both the abscissa and the ordinate have been scaled to take account of each observer's grating resolution. Results from normal eyes shown by the dotted line. Results from anisometropic amblyopes shown by open symbols. Results from strabismic amblyopes shown by filled symbols. Vernier acuity, when scaled like this, is close to normal for anisometropic amblyopes, and far from normal for strabismic amblyopes. Reprinted with permission from Levi, D. M., and Klein, S., 1982, Hyperacuity and amblyopia, *Nature* **298**:268–270. Copyright 1982, MacMillan Magazines Limited.

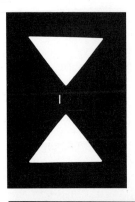

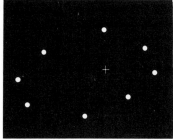

FIG. 8.13. (Top) Spatial localization task. The subject is asked to line up the line between the points of the two triangles. (Bottom) Spatial distortion in a strabismic amblyope. The subject set the dots to be equidistant from the central cross. The rightmost dot was 1.5° from the cross. Reprinted with permission from Flom, M. C., and Bedell, H. E., 1985, Identifying amblyopia using associated conditions, acuity, and nonacuity features, *Am. J. Optom. Physiol. Opt.* 62:153–160.

anisometropic amblyopes can be accounted for by their contrast sensitivity deficit (Hess and Holliday, 1992), both spatial uncertainty and vernier acuity are distinctly worse in strabismic amblyopes than their contrast sensitivity deficit would predict.

IV. The Peripheral Part of the Field of View

Physicians are concerned primarily with acuity in the central part of the field of view. The aim is to get the two eyes to look in the same direction in order to avoid double vision. This requires the establishment of the fovea as the fixation point, which in turn requires improvement of acuity in the foveal region until it is as close as possible as normal. Yet strabismus leads to mismatches in the images in the peripheral part of the retina as well as in the center, and anisometropia, if severe, leads to blurring of the image that is significant in the peripheral part of the retina as well as the center. Very few studies have considered this question.

Acuity is reduced out to 20° from the fovea in strabismic amblyopes (Sireteanu and Fronius, 1981). There is considerable variability in the extent of the deficit in this region from one case to another (Hess and Jacobs, 1979; see Fig. 8.14). Generally speaking, acuity is reduced more in the nasal part of the retina for esotropes, and in the temporal part of the retina for exotropes. This is the part of the retina that is closer to the fovea, and therefore the mismatch between the two images is likely to have more effect there, because the size of the receptive fields of the cells involved is smaller. Anisometropic amblyopes have

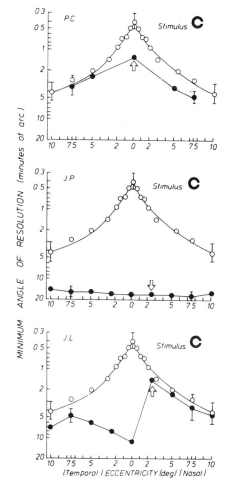

FIG. 8.14. Acuity as a function of eccentricity in three strabismic amblyopes. Open circles represent the acuity from four normal subjects. Filled circles show the acuity from the amblyopes. Arrow marks the point of fixation. Amblyope PC had central fixation, and a small symmetric reduction in acuity. Amblyope JP had fixation 2° away from the fovea, and a large reduction in acuity at all eccentricities. Amblyope JL was an exotrope, and acuity was reduced substantially more in the temporal field of view than in the nasal. Reprinted with kind permission from Hess, R. F., and Jacobs, R. J., 1979, A preliminary report of acuity and contour interaction across the amblyope's visual field, *Vision Res.* **19**:1403–1408. Copyright 1979, Elsevier Science, Ltd., The Boulevard, Langford Lane, Kidlington OX5 1GB, UK.

reduced acuity over a wider area of retina than strabismic amblyopes. Somehow, the diffusion of the image is a stronger influence than the lateral displacement of the image on cells with large receptive fields at large eccentricities.

Binocular interaction has been studied in the peripheral part of the field of view in amblyopes with tests of binocular summation, and transfer of the "tilt after-effect" (Sireteanu *et al.*, 1981). Generally, results from these tests were deficient in the areas of reduced acuity. That is, binocular interactions were present in the peripheral part of the field of view of strabismic amblyopes, but not for anisometropic amblyopes. However, the results varied considerably from case to case, depending on the extent of the amblyopia.

There can also be interesting variations in retinal correspondence between center and periphery of the field of view. The easiest to explain occurs in strabismics with a large angle of deviation, which is too large to get anomalous retinal correspondence in the central part of the field of view. Compensation in this part of the field of view occurs through suppression of the image in the deviating eye. However, anomalous retinal correspondence may occur in the *peripheral* part of the field of view, where the receptive fields of cells are larger, and the anatomical distance in the cortex over which connections must be rearranged to get anomalous correspondence is smaller (Sireteanu and Fronius, 1989). As a result, subjective localization in the central part of the field of view differs in the two eyes, whereas subjective localization in the peripheral part of the field of view is the same (Fig. 8.15).

The general conclusion is that the reduction in acuity depends on the extent of the binocular mismatch in relation to the size of the receptive fields of the part of the retina involved. A moderate mismatch will have a large effect where the receptive fields are small, near the fovea, and a small effect where the receptive fields are large, in the periphery. Binocular interactions are affected similarly to acuity. In some cases, acuity, binocular interactions, and subjective localization are all degraded severely near the fovea, yet are normal in the peripheral part of the field of view.

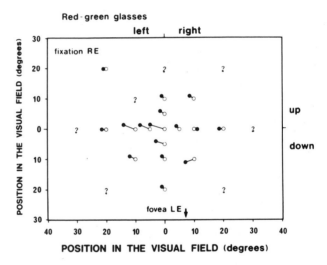

FIG. 8.15. Subjective localization by an untreated strabismic amblyope. Red stimulus presented to one eye, and green stimulus to the other through red-green glasses. (O) Normal eye; (●) amblyopic eye; (?) decision about the relative localization of the stimuli was not possible. Reprinted with permission from *Investigative Ophthalmology and Visual Science*, Sireteanu and Fronius (1989).

V. Summary

Amblyopia includes a variety of deficits. In nearly all cases there is a loss of acuity and contrast sensitivity, although in two cases described by Hess, Campbell, and Greenhalgh this was not true. Vernier acuity is degraded. Spatial localization is distorted. The details of objects are distorted.

In anisometropia, most of these factors are degraded in proportion to each other. Vernier acuity and Snellen acuity are reduced in proportion to the loss of resolution measured by grating acuity. Spatial uncertainty can be explained by the loss of contrast sensitivity. In strabismus, vernier acuity and Snellen acuity are reduced more than grating acuity. If the angle of deviation of the eye is constant and not too large, there will be a new point of fixation. In this case, vision will be clearest in the peripheral part of the field of view in the direction of the fovea. If the angle of deviation is large, the image in one eye will be suppressed, because it is not possible for the anatomical connections to be rearranged over the large distance required to compensate for the deficit. In bilateral cataract, the result is like a bad case of anisometropia. In unilateral cataract, the situation is much worse: spatial vision is almost totally lost in one eye.

There have been discussions in the literature as to whether amblyopia is caused by loss of connections between retina and cortex (undersampling), blurring of these connections (spatial uncertainty), or rearrangement of these connections (spatial scrambling) (Levi and Klein, 1990; Hess et al., 1990; Wilson, 1991). It should be clear from this chapter that all three occur in different forms of amblyopia, and all three could occur in a single case of amblyopia. The clearest case of loss of connections between retina and cortex is in monocular deprivation, or stimulus deprivation amblyopia, where these connections are radically reduced. However, some reduction in strength of connections has been documented in animal models of anisometropia and strabismus. From an anatomical point of view, blurring of connections and rearrangement of connections are the same fundamental phenomenon. It is just a question of whether the connections are rearranged in a circularly symmetric fashion, as in anisometropia, or in a bipolar fashion, as in anomalous retinal correspondence from strabismus, or something in between. It seems likely that, in severe cases of strabismus with anomalous retinal correspondence, several forms of rearrangement will occur: formation of two sets of connections between retina and cortex, one from the new point of fixation to central vision, and one from the new point of fixation to its normal location; a blurring of the precise topography around each of these locations; and some loss in the density of the connections from the amblyopic eye. In addition to these various forms of anatomical rearrangement, there is also the physiological suppression of the image in the amblyopic eye by the image in the normal eye.

The variety of results that can occur is illustrated clearly in the classic paper of Hess et al. (1978). What this paper also illustrates is that measurement of the contrast sensitivity curve can obscure the details of the loss of vision in the patient. The contrast sensitivity curve lumps together a number of different conditions, because the stimulus covers a wide area of retina, and the patient detects the grating on the basis of whatever part of the retina has the most distinct vision. Moreover, the contrast sensitivity curve does not detect errors in spatial localization. To understand the full nature of the deficit, a variety of tests have to be performed.

References

Bradley, A., and Freeman, R. D., 1981, Contrast sensitivity in anisometropic amblyopia, *Invest. Ophthalmol. Vis. Sci.* **21**:467–476.

Enoch, J. M., Berger, R., and Birns, R., 1970, A static perimetric technique believed to test receptive field properties: Extension and verification of the analysis, *Doc. Ophthalmol.* **29**:127–153.

Flom, M. C., and Bedell, H. E., 1985, Identifying amblyopia using associated conditions, acuity, and nonacuity features, *Am. J. Optom. Physiol. Opt.* **62:**153–160.

Flom, M. C., Weymouth, F. W., and Kahneman, D., 1963, Visual resolution and contour interaction, *J. Opt. Soc. Am. [A]* **53:**1026–1032.

Gstalder, R. J., and Green, D. G., 1971, Laser interferometric acuity in amblyopia, *J. Pediatr. Ophthalmol.* **8:**251–256.

Hess, R. F., 1977, On the relationship between strabismic amblyopia and eccentric fixation, *Br. J. Ophthalmol.* **61:**767–773.

Hess, R. F., and Holliday, I. E., 1992, The spatial localization deficit in amblyopia, *Vision Res.* **32:**1319–1339.

Hess, R. F., and Jacobs, R. J., 1979, A preliminary report of acuity and contour interaction across the amblyope's visual field, *Vision Res.* **19:**1403–1408.

Hess, R. F., and Pointer, J. S., 1985, Differences in the neural basis of human amblyopia: The distribution of the anomaly across the visual field, *Vision Res.* **25:**1577–1594.

Hess, R. F., Campbell, F. W., and Greenhalgh, T., 1978, On the nature of the neural abnormality in human amblyopia: Neural aberrations and neural sensitivity loss, *Pfluegers Arch. Gesamte Physiol.* **377:**201–207.

Hess, R. F., Field, D. J., and Watt, R. J., 1990, The puzzle of amblyopia, in: *Vision: Coding and Efficiency* (C. Blakemore, ed.), Cambridge University Press, London.

Hubel, D. H., and Wiesel, T. N., 1960, Receptive fields of optic nerve fibres in the spider monkey, *J. Physiol. (London)* **154:**572–580.

Irvine, S. R., 1948, Amblyopia ex anopsia. Observations on retinal inhibition, scotoma, projection, light difference discrimination and visual acuity, *Trans. Am. Ophthalmol. Soc.* **66:**527–575.

Katz, B., and Sireteanu, R., 1990, The Teller acuity card test: A useful method for the clinical routine? *Clin. Vis. Sci.* **5:**307–323.

Levi, D. M., and Klein, S., 1982, Hyperacuity and amblyopia, *Nature* **298:**268–270.

Levi, D. M., and Klein, S. A., 1985, Vernier acuity, crowding and amblyopia, *Vision Res.* **25:**979–991.

Levi, D. M., and Klein, S. A., 1990, Equivalent intrinsic blur in amblyopia, *Vision Res.* **30:**1995–2022.

Maurer, D., and Lewis, T. L., 1993, Visual outcomes after infantile cataract, in: *Early Visual Development, Normal and Abnormal* (K. Simons, ed.), Oxford University Press, London, pp. 454–484.

Pugh, M., 1962, Amblyopia and the retina, *Br. J. Ophthalmol.* **46:**193–211.

Sireteanu, R., and Fronius, M., 1981, Naso-temporal asymmetries in human amblyopia: Consequence of long-term interocular suppression, *Vision Res.* **21:**1055–1063.

Sireteanu, R., and Fronius, M., 1989, Different patterns of retinal correspondence in the central and peripheral visual field of strabismics, *Invest. Ophthalmol. Vis. Sci.* **30:**2023–2033.

Sireteanu, R., Fronius, M., and Singer, W., 1981, Binocular interaction in the peripheral visual field of humans with strabismic and anisometropic amblyopia, *Vision Res.* **21:**1065–1074.

Stuart, J. A., and Burian, H. M., 1962, A study of separation difficulty, *Am. J. Ophthalmol.* **53:**471–477.

Wilson, H. R., 1991, Model of peripheral and amblyopic hyperacuity, *Vision Res.* **31:**967–982.

9

Critical Periods

We have known for several decades that visual deprivation affects infants more than adults. Children can compensate for strabismus, anisometropia, and cataract before the age of 7. They can also compensate for any surgery or optical corrections that change the image on the retina back to normal. There is a period of time during development, known as the critical period, during which the anatomy and physiology of the visual system are mutable, or plastic. However, once the critical period is past, compensation for visual deprivation rarely occurs.

I. General Principles from Experiments with Animals

The critical period that has been most carefully characterized is the critical period for monocular deprivation in the cat. The visual cortex is very susceptible to the closure of one eye between 4 and 6 weeks of age (Hubel and Wiesel, 1970). At that age, closure of one eye for 3 days leads to a cortex in which most cells are dominated by the open eye. Susceptibility to deprivation then declines between 6 weeks and 3 months of age. Some susceptibility remains until 8–9 months of age (Daw et al., 1992; see Fig. 9.1). The critical period for ocular dominance changes in strabismus has a similar time course (Levitt and Van Sluyters, 1982).

The critical period depends on the level of the visual system that is being studied. Cells in layer IV (the input layer) are less likely to have their ocular dominance altered than cells in layers II, III, V, and VI (the output layers) at all ages (Shatz and Stryker, 1978; Mower et al., 1985). It is not clear if the critical period ends earlier in layer IV than in other layers, or if the susceptibility in layer IV just drops to insignificant levels (Daw et al., 1992), but the result is effectively the same: late in the critical period, layers II, III, V, and VI are noticeably plastic, while layer IV is not.

The visual system is more plastic, and remains plastic for a longer period of time, at higher levels of processing (see Daw, 1994). The retina is largely hard-wired at birth (Sherman and Stone, 1973). There is some plasticity in the lateral geniculate nucleus, but not much (see Sherman, 1985). The output layers of primary visual cortex are more plastic than the input layers. Visual cortex

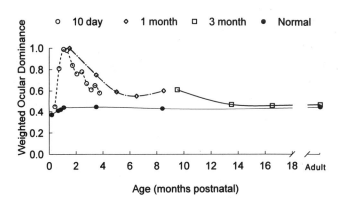

FIG. 9.1. Critical period for monocular deprivation in the cat. Weighted ocular dominance is calculated as $n_7 + {}^5\!/\!_6 n_6 + {}^4\!/\!_6 n_5 + {}^3\!/\!_6 n_4 + {}^2\!/\!_6 n_3 + {}^1\!/\!_6 n_2$, where n_i is the number of cells in ocular dominance group i, divided by the total number of cells recorded. Weighted ocular dominance for normal animals is 0.43, because there is a slight dominance by the contralateral eye. Points for 10 days of deprivation from Olson and Freeman (1980); for 1 month from Jones *et al.* (1984); for 3 months from Daw *et al.* (1992). Reprinted with permission from *Investigative Ophthalmology and Visual Science*, Daw (1994).

projects to inferior temporal cortex, where faces and objects are recognized, and plasticity continues for a substantial period of time (Rodman, 1994). Visual memories are also stored in temporal cortex, and plasticity presumably continues for them indefinitely. Temporal cortex projects to the hippocampus, which is known to be plastic in the adult.

There are also different critical periods for different visual properties. This is most clearly illustrated by a comparison of the critical period for direction selectivity, and the critical period for ocular dominance in the cat. The critical period for direction selectivity is half over at 4 weeks of age, and substantially finished at 6 weeks of age, when the critical period for ocular dominance changes is still at its peak (Daw and Wyatt, 1976; see Fig. 9.2). As a demonstration of this point, one can rear cats in a visual environment moving right, with the right eye open until 5 weeks of age, then switch them to an environment moving left, with the left eye open. The result is a cortex in which most direction-selective cells prefer rightward movement, and are dominated by the left eye, because the switch occurred when the critical period for direction selectivity was largely over, but the critical period for eye dominance was at its height (Daw *et al.*, 1978). Results from both cat and ferret also show that orientation selectivity develops in layer IV before ocular dominance segregation (Chapman and Stryker, 1993; Kim and Bonhoeffer, 1993). This result fits in with the general point that critical periods are later for higher levels of processing: the input layer of primary visual cortex, layer IV, is a lower level of processing than the output layers II, III, V, and VI, and direction and orientation selectivity are properties of the input layer whereas binocularity is more a property of the output layers (Shatz and Stryker, 1978).

Interestingly, switching from one eye open to the other eye open (reverse suture) in the monkey shows that the critical period in the visual cortex for the magnocellular system ends earlier than the critical period for the parvocellular

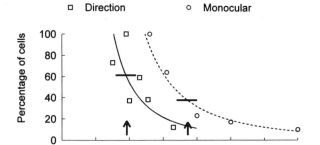

FIG. 9.2. Comparison of critical periods for direction-selective and ocular dominance changes. Animals were reared in one condition (right eye open, or environment moving right) and then switched to the opposite (left eye open or movement left) at an age that varied from animal to animal. Points plot the percentage of cells preferring the direction seen second, or the eye open second. The curve for direction-selective changes passes through the normal ratio (60%) before 4 weeks of age, and the curve for ocular dominance changes passes through the normal ratio (43%) after 7 weeks of age. Points from Blakemore and Van Sluyters (1974) and Daw and Wyatt (1976). Reprinted with permission from *Investigative Ophthalmology and Visual Science*, Daw (1994).

system (LeVay *et al.*, 1980). The parvocellular layers of the lateral geniculate project to layer IVCβ, while the magnocellular layers project to layer IVCα. When reverse suture is done at 3 weeks of age, the eye open second can reverse the effects of the initial deprivation in the cortical layer for the parvocellular system (IVCβ), but not in the cortical layer for the magnocellular system (IVCα) (Fig. 9.3). Presumably connections for movement need to be wired into place while connections for fine acuity continue to develop.

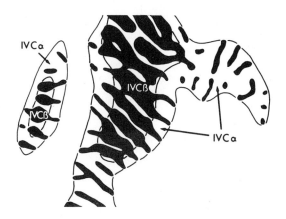

FIG. 9.3. Effect of reverse suture at 3 weeks of age on labeling pattern in the right cortex. Right eye sutured first, then opened and left eye sutured. Right eye was injected. Right eye (black area) dominated in layer IVCβ because this layer was still plastic at 3 weeks of age; left eye (white area) dominated in layer IVCα, because the critical period for this layer was over at 3 weeks of age. Reprinted with permission from LeVay, S., Wiesel, T. N., and Hubel, D. H., 1980, The development of ocular dominance columns in normal and visually deprived monkeys, *J. Comp. Neurol.* **191:**1–51. Copyright 1980, John Wiley & Sons, Inc.

Monocular deprivation can be used to compare critical periods in different species. The critical period for monocular deprivation in the cat starts at 3 weeks of age, a little after the eyes open. In the macaque monkey, the eyes are open at birth, and the animal is susceptible to ocular dominance shifts soon after birth. The peak of this critical period is around 1 month of age (LeVay *et al.*, 1980). The end is a little after 1 year of age. In humans, very substantial effects from unilateral cataract are seen at any time between birth and 3 years of age (Vaegan and Taylor, 1979; see Fig. 9.4). Some susceptibility remains until 8– 9 years of age. The general conclusion is that, in all three species, the critical period for ocular dominance changes starts soon after the eyes open, and continues until some time near puberty.

The timing of the peak of the critical period for ocular dominance changes is significant. It occurs while ocular dominance columns in layer IV are segregating, and cells sensitive to disparity are being formed. As described in Chapter 3, these two events are correlated with each other in cat, monkey, and human. This period is a crucial one for the development of binocular vision. As the left and right eye inputs to layer IV in primary visual cortex segregate, cells

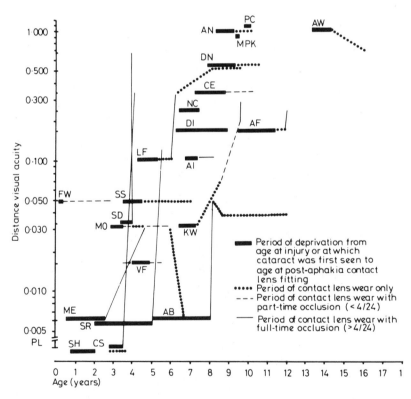

FIG. 9.4. Cases of unilateral cataract in man, in which the beginning and end of deprivation are well defined. Heavy horizontal bars span the period of deprivation and are set at the level of the first visual acuity score obtained after adequate correction after taking out the cataract. Lighter lines show subsequent responses to various treatments. Reprinted with permission from Vaegen and Taylor, 1979, *Trans. Ophthalmol. Soc. UK* **99**:432–439. (Published by BMJ Publishing Group.)

sensitive to disparity are formed at higher levels of the system, and cells in all layers are most susceptible to alterations in the input from one eye as compared to the other. This crucial period is at 4–6 weeks in the cat, around 1 month in the macaque, and 3–5 months in humans.

We can now propose a rationale about why orientation and direction selectivity develop earlier than ocular dominance. Disparity-sensitive cells need to have input from cells that have coordinated direction and orientation selectivity in left and right eyes (Daw, 1994): it would not make any sense for a disparity-selective cell to have input for vertical lines from one eye, and input for horizontal lines from the other. During the prestereoptic period, the direction and orientation tuning of cells in layer IV becomes tighter, while the cells are still binocular. Then, after the columns for direction and orientation have been tightly organized, cells in layer IV become monocular, and provide inputs to disparity-sensitive cells which correlate them. Thus, the critical period for direction selectivity ends at the time when stereoscopic acuity is rising rapidly, and cells are very sensitive to ocular dominance changes (Fig. 9.5).

Monocular deprivation has an effect on a variety of functions besides ocular dominance, and the critical period for these varies (Harwerth et al., 1986; see Fig. 9.6). Monkeys with one eye sutured have their sensitivity to light reduced in the dark-adapted state, if the suture is done before 3 months of age, but not afterward. In the light-adapted state, their sensitivity to increments above the background is reduced, and the spectral sensitivity curve is altered. This occurs for deprivation before 6 months of age, but not afterward. Deficits in the high-frequency part of the contrast sensitivity curve are found with deprivations up to 18 months of age. Binocular summation is disturbed, even if deprivation is delayed to 25 months of age. The order of these sensitive periods also makes the point that functions requiring higher levels of processing have later sensitive periods.

These results show that some functions remain plastic until a late stage of life. Indeed, some manipulations have an effect in the adult (Gilbert and Wie-

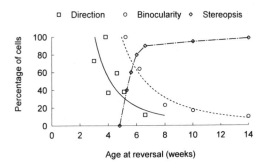

FIG. 9.5. Comparison of the decline in sensitivity to direction changes with the increase in sensitivity to stereopsis, and the decline in sensitivity to ocular dominance changes in the cat. At 5 weeks of age, cells are not very susceptible to direction changes. Between 5 and 6 weeks of age, cells are very sensitive to ocular dominance changes, and ability to discriminate stereoscopic targets increases rapidly. After 6 weeks of age, a substantial sensitivity to ocular dominance changes remains. Reprinted with permission from *Investigative Ophthalmology and Visual Science*, Daw (1994).

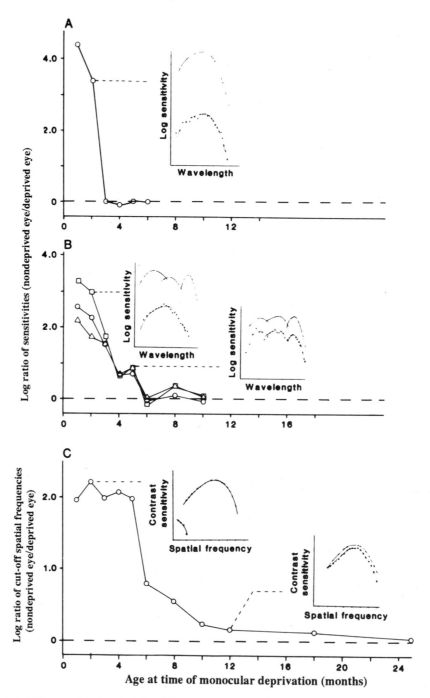

FIG. 9.6. Different critical periods for different functions in the macaque monkey. (A) Comparison of the dark-adapted (scotopic) spectral sensitivity in the two eyes, for deprivations starting at various ages. (B) Comparison of the light-adapted (photopic) spectral sensitivity in the two eyes. (C) Comparison of contrast sensitivity curves in the two eyes. Reprinted with permission from Harwerth *et al.*, *Science* **232**:235–237. Copyright 1986, American Association for the Advancement of Science.

sel, 1992): if large lesions are made with a laser in the retinas of both eyes, so that the cortex has no sensory input from this area, cells in the cortex representing the area of the lesion will start responding to areas in the retina outside the lesion. There is a short-term physiological change, and also a long-term anatomical change occurring over a period of months, through sprouting of lateral connections in the cortex (Darian-Smith and Gilbert, 1994). The physiological changes can be produced with an artificial scotoma as well as a lesion (Pettet and Gilbert, 1992).

These results show that the critical period depends on the severity of the alteration in the periphery. Lesions are a more drastic manipulation than alterations of the optics of the eye. Injection of tetrodotoxin into the eye, which abolishes activity altogether, is known to have a more powerful effect than rearing in the dark, which produces a reduced and disorganized level of activity (Stryker and Harris, 1986). This point is emphasized by cases of amblyopia in humans, where loss of the good eye in teenagers and adults can lead to a dramatic improvement in acuity in the amblyopic eye (Vereecken and Brabant, 1984) even at the age of 65 when patching of the good eye is known to be useless (Tierney, 1989).

The critical period for the development of amblyopia is best studied in primates, which have a fovea. Their acuity varies with eccentricity much more dramatically than it does in the cat. The situation is complicated, because no study of the critical period has been done for anisometropia, and there are a number of factors that can affect the results in strabismus (Kiorpes et al., 1989). Unfortunately, no study has yet been completed on the effect of a fixed period of strabismus at a variety of ages, because a very large number of experiments need to be done to get a significant number of results with the angle of deviation the same from animal to animal. Moreover, two sets of animals need to be studied: some with small angles of deviation, leading to a new point of fixation, and others with a large angle of deviation, leading to suppression of the image in one eye and/or alternate fixation. In naturally strabismic monkeys, acuity develops more slowly than it does in normal monkeys (graphs comparing their acuity diverge at 5–10 weeks of age), and the final acuity is significantly worse than normal (Kiorpes, 1989; see Fig. 9.7). Reductions in acuity are found in both eyes. The general conclusion is that monkeys are susceptible to strabismus

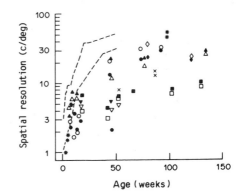

FIG. 9.7. Development of spatial resolution in naturally strabismic monkeys. Open symbols represent right eye data, and closed symbols left eye data. Dashed lines represent range of visual resolution for 38 normal monkeys. Reprinted with kind permission from Kiorpes, L., 1989, The development of spatial resolution and contrast sensitivity in naturally strabismic monkeys, Br. J. Ophthalmol. 4:279–293. Copyright 1989, Elsevier Science, Ltd., The Boulevard, Langford Lane, Kidlington OX5 1GB, UK.

between birth and 10 weeks of age, but when the critical period comes to an end is unknown.

II. The Critical Period in Humans

General experience in the clinic is that children are susceptible to optical and motor problems until the age of 7 or 8 years (von Noorden, 1990). However, the situation is complicated by the number of different deficits that can occur, and the number of functions that can be measured: acuity, contrast sensitivity, binocularity, stereopsis, and others. Moreover, the extent of the deficit may be quite variable over the first few years of life. The clinician will try to rectify the deficit soon after seeing it, and reports of the extent and nature of the deficit before the clinician sees it are, in general, not very accurate. In other words, most studies are retrospective, and where there are prospective studies, therapy starts as soon as it is known to be effective.

Few deficits lead to amblyopia before 6 months of age. Children are frequently born with astigmatism, which goes away over the first 6 months without permanent harm. Astigmatism leads to meridional amblyopia only if it persists for 2 years or more (see Atkinson, 1993). Anisometropia may be associated with the astigmatism, and again, only anisometropia persistent for 3 years or more leads to deficits (Abrahamsson et al., 1990). Anisometropia that is persistent between 3 months and several years of life seems to be quite rare (Almeder et al., 1990). Consequently, it is hard to say exactly what the critical period for amblyopia is, in cases of pure anisometropia that are not associated with strabismus. However, the general rule seems to be that astigmatism and anisometropia need to be persistent for 2 years or more from an early age to lead to a permanent deficit in acuity.

Cataract and other forms of stimulus deprivation have a much more severe effect than anisometropia or astigmatism. The critical period for the effect of these three conditions on acuity is probably much the same (see Fig. 9.4). However, because the effect is more severe in stimulus deprivation, much shorter periods of deprivation have a profound effect. Occlusion for 1–2 weeks before the age of 18 months has a substantial effect, although the cause is often complicated, because many such patients develop strabismus after their operation (Awaya et al., 1979). In congenital cases, best results are obtained if surgery is done in the first few months of life, and is followed by aggressive therapy (Birch et al., 1986; Maurer and Lewis, 1993; see Fig. 9.8). A contact lens or spectacle correction for the eye lacking a lens will produce an image that is different in size from the image in the normal eye (aniseikonia). An intraocular lens implant or glasses that compensate for the difference in magnification produce a better result if the infant will tolerate them (Enoch and Rabinowicz, 1976). The overall conclusion is that weeks of deprivation have a substantial effect between 6 and 18 months of age, and months of deprivation can have an effect until 8 years of age.

With strabismic patients one needs to consider amblyopia, binocular function, and stereopsis. Amblyopia does not develop in congenital esotropia until close to 1 year of age. Birch and Stager (1985) studied the difference in acuity

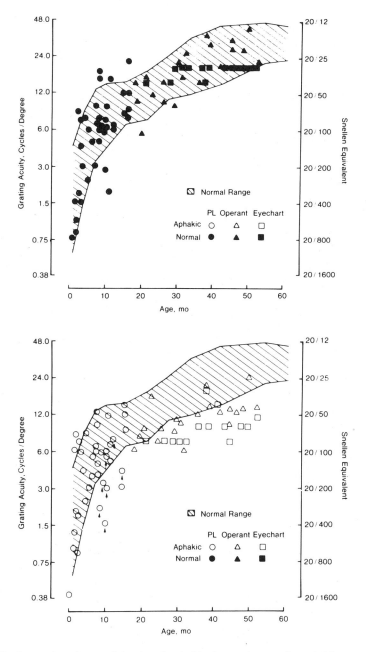

FIG. 9.8. Grating acuity of normal (top) and aphakic (bottom) eyes of 16 children aged 1 to 53 months, compared to the normal range. Reprinted with permission from Birch, E. E., Stager, D. R., and Wright, W. W., *Arch. Ophthalmol.* **104:**1783–1787. Copyright 1986, American Medical Association.

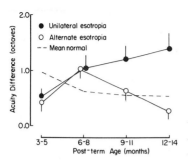

FIG. 9.9. Acuity difference between the two eyes for normal infants, and untreated esotropes, either unilateral or alternating. The acuity difference does not go significantly outside the normal range for unilateral esotropes until near 1 year of age. Reprinted with permission from *Investigative Ophthalmology and Visual Science*, Birch and Stager (1985).

between the two eyes for unilateral esotropes, and found that it did not go significantly outside the normal range until 9–11 months (Fig. 9.9). Children seem to be particularly susceptible at this age: one infant who developed esotropia at 10 months of age had a loss of acuity after only 4 weeks (Jacobson *et al.*, 1981). There can definitely be a loss of acuity from strabismus after 1 year of age, when acuity in normal children reaches levels close to the adult level. Deficits can occur up to the age of 8 years. Probably the period of peak sensitivity lies between 9 months and 2 years of age, and sensitivity declines between 2 and 8 years of age, but there are no hard numbers that provide a quantitative measurement of this (von Noorden, 1990). Unfortunately, one is faced in strabismus with the problem that the extent of the deviation may be variable, and that amblyopia will depend on the magnitude of the deviation, in addition to the problem that most clinical studies are retrospective.

Binocular function can be measured in a variety of ways. One way is to observe interocular transfer of the "tilt aftereffect" (Banks *et al.*, 1975; Hohmann and Creutzfeldt, 1975). In the tilt aftereffect, a subject stares at a set of lines tilted to the left, and then observes a set of vertical lines, which appear to be tilted to the right. One can measure the extent of the effect, by showing the subject lines that are not quite vertical, and observing how far they have to be tilted to compensate for the aftereffect. Interocular transfer is measured by looking at the initial display with one eye, and comparing the extent of the aftereffect in that eye with the aftereffect in the other eye. Interocular transfer is a measure of the percentage of cells in the visual cortex that receive binocular input. Modeling of the results suggests that the critical period starts between birth and 6 months of age, peaks at 1–2 years of age, and declines between 1–2 and 8 years of age (Fig. 9.10).

Stereopsis can be found in untreated esotropes, although their stereoscopic acuity is substantially below adult levels. After the deviation is corrected at an early age with prisms, 50% have stereopsis at 3–5 months of age, and the percentage drops substantially by 6–8 months of age (Birch and Stager, 1985; see Fig. 9.11). Coarse stereopsis may be present up to 2½ years of age (Mohindra *et al.*, 1985), although the extent of the stereopsis depends on the criteria used to measure it (Dobson and Sebris, 1989). No study has measured stereoscopic acuity, because of the time and effort required, so there is no quantitative measure of the extent of stereopsis in any of the studies. In general, the prospective studies, using forced choice preferential looking, have confirmed the clini-

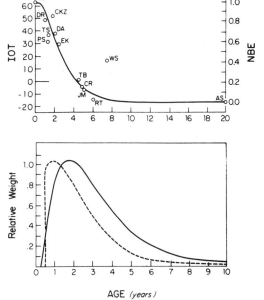

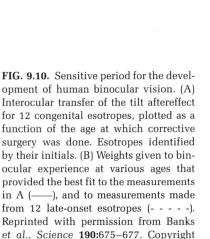

FIG. 9.10. Sensitive period for the development of human binocular vision. (A) Interocular transfer of the tilt aftereffect for 12 congenital esotropes, plotted as a function of the age at which corrective surgery was done. Esotropes identified by their initials. (B) Weights given to binocular experience at various ages that provided the best fit to the measurements in A (——), and to measurements made from 12 late-onset esotropes (- - - - -). Reprinted with permission from Banks *et al., Science* **190:**675–677. Copyright 1975, American Association for the Advancement of Science.

cal experience that alignment before 1½ years combined with exercises can give crude stereopsis, but alignment after that time does not (Jampolsky, 1978).

One of the therapies for amblyopia is to patch the good eye. Given that monocular deprivation has a stronger effect than any other form of deprivation, this can be a dangerous procedure: the acuity in the good eye can be reduced (Odom *et al.*, 1982). Total patching of the good eye can therefore lead to reversed amblyopia or even bilateral amblyopia. Experiments with cats show that bilateral amblyopia can be avoided, if the good eye is patched 50–70% of the time, and both eyes are open part of the time (Mitchell, 1991). This confirms clinical experience (von Noorden, 1990; Maurer and Lewis, 1993). As discussed above, reasonable acuity can be achieved in both eyes, and some form of binocular vision, but there will be no stereopsis unless the eyes are aligned, binocular fusion is achieved, and exercises are started well before 18 months to 2 years of age.

The general rule is that none of the deficits discussed—strabismus, anisometropia, astigmatism, or even cataract—will lead to amblyopia if they oc-

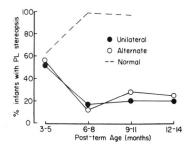

FIG. 9.11. Percentage of normal and esotropic children who reached criterion for demonstrating stereopsis using a static stereogram, and preferential looking. Reprinted with permission from *Investigative Ophthalmology and Visual Science*, Birch and Stager (1985).

cur after the age of 8 years. However, a deficit that is created before the age of 8 years can be at least partly corrected afterward. There are numerous reports in the literature of success in reducing amblyopia in teenagers (Birnbaum *et al.*, 1977). Thus, the critical period for cure of amblyopia lasts longer than the critical period for its creation. However, this may not be true of stereopsis. It is hard to get any stereopsis back after 18 months of age if it is destroyed before this time, but stereopsis can clearly be reduced even after 18 months of age. Part of the reason for this difference may be that stereopsis is degraded by a reduction in acuity in everybody, including normal people. Consequently, amblyopia appearing after 18 months of age will automatically lead to a degradation of stereopsis.

III. Summary

We can now relate critical periods for the effects of deprivation to the various stages in the development of the visual system discussed in Chapter 3. There are three periods in the development of the visual system: prestereoptic (0–4 months in humans), onset of stereopsis (4–6 months), and poststereoptic (6 months–2 years). In the prestereoptic period, acuity develops and direction and orientation specificity are refined. Stereoscopic acuity then goes from nil to near adult levels in a period of 1 month at the same time that ocular dominance columns segregate. In the poststereoptic period, acuity continues to develop for another year.

These functions are all plastic for a period after they first develop. A reduction in amblyopia can occur after 2 years, up to 8 years of age. Binocular function can be disrupted up to 8 years of age, and stereopsis is affected particularly between 6 and 18 months of age. The critical period for direction selectivity in the human is not known, but meridional amblyopia can certainly occur from astigmatism after 6 months of age; indeed, it never occurs before. A parallel general principle is found in animals, where monocular deprivation has an effect for some period of time after the ocular dominance columns first form.

Another general principle is that functions dealt with at a higher level of the system have a later critical period. The sequence, going from lower levels to higher levels, is dark-adapted sensitivity, light-adapted sensitivity, direction selectivity, acuity, and ocular dominance. Where stereopsis fits into this sequence is not completely clear: the situation is complicated by the interaction between stereopsis and acuity, which occurs in both normal and deprived people, and consequently stereopsis may be an exception to this rule.

Finally, at least for amblyopia, the critical period for a cure lasts longer than the critical period for creation of a deficit.

References

Abrahamsson, M., Fabian, G., and Sjostrand, J., 1990, A longitudinal study of a population based sample of astigmatic children. II. The changeability of anisometropia, *Acta Ophthalmol.* **68**:435–440.

Almeder, L. M., Peck, L. B., and Howland, H. C., 1990, Prevalence of anisometropia in volunteer laboratory and school screening populations, *Invest. Ophthalmol. Vis. Sci.* **31**:2448–2455.

Atkinson, J., 1993, Infant vision screening: Prediction and prevention of strabismus and amblyopia from refractive screening in the Cambridge photorefraction program, in: *Early Visual Development, Normal and Abnormal* (K. Simons, ed.), Oxford University Press, London, pp. 335–348.

Awaya, S., Sugawara, M., and Miyake, S., 1979, Observations in patients with occlusion amblyopia, *Trans. Ophthalmol. Soc. U.K.* **99**:447–454.

Banks, M. S., Aslin, R. N., and Letson, R. D., 1975, Sensitive period for the development of human binocular vision, *Science* **190**:675–677.

Birch, E. E., and Stager, D. R., 1985, Monocular acuity and stereopsis in infantile esotropia, *Invest. Ophthalmol. Vis. Sci.* **26**:1624–1630.

Birch, E. E., Stager, D. R., and Wright, W. W., 1986, Grating acuity development after early surgery for congenital unilateral cataract, *Arch. Ophthalmol.* **104**:1783–1787.

Birnbaum, M. H., Koslowe, K., and Sanet, R., 1977, Success in amblyopia therapy as a function of age: A literature survey, *Arch. Ophthalmol.* **54**:269–275.

Blakemore, C., and Van Sluyters, R. C., 1974, Reversal of the physiological effects of monocular deprivation in kittens: Further evidence for a sensitive period, *J. Physiol. (London)* **237**:195–216.

Chapman, B., and Stryker, M. P., 1993, Development of orientation selectivity in ferret visual cortex and effects of deprivation, *J. Neurosci.* **13**:5251–5262.

Darian-Smith, C., and Gilbert, C. D., 1994, Axonal sprouting accompanies functional reorganization in adult cat striate cortex, *Nature* **368**:737–740.

Daw, N. W., 1994, Mechanisms of plasticity in the visual cortex, *Invest. Ophthalmol. Vis. Sci.* **35**:4168–4179.

Daw, N. W., and Wyatt, H. J., 1976, Kittens reared in a unidirectional environment: Evidence for a critical period, *J. Physiol. (London)* **257**:155–170.

Daw, N. W., Berman, N. E. J., and Ariel, M., 1978, Interaction of critical periods in the visual cortex of kittens, *Science* **199**:565–567.

Daw, N. W., Fox, K., Sato, H., and Czepita, D., 1992, Critical period for monocular deprivation in the cat visual cortex, *J. Neurophysiol.* **67**:197–202.

Dobson, V., and Sebris, S. L., 1989, Longitudinal study of acuity and stereopsis in infants with or at-risk for esotropia, *Invest. Ophthalmol. Vis. Sci.* **30**:1146–1158.

Enoch, J. M., and Rabinowicz, I. M., 1976, Early surgery and visual correction of an infant born with unilateral lens opacity, *Doc. Ophthalmol.* **41**:371–382.

Gilbert, C. D., and Wiesel, T. N., 1992, Receptive field dynamics in adult primary visual cortex, *Nature* **356**:150–152.

Harwerth, R. S., Smith, E. L., Duncan, G. C., Crawford, M. L. J., and von Noorden, G. K., 1986, Multiple sensitive periods in the development of the primate visual system, *Science* **232**:235–238.

Hohmann, A., and Creutzfeldt, O. D., 1975, Squint and the development of binocularity in humans, *Nature* **254**:613–614.

Hubel, D. H., and Wiesel, T. N., 1970, The period of susceptibility to the physiological effects of unilateral eye closure in kittens, *J. Physiol. (London)* **206**:419–436.

Jacobson, S., Mohindra, I., and Held, R., 1981, Age of onset of amblyopia in infants with esotropia, *Doc. Ophthalmol.* **30**:210–216.

Jampolsky, A., 1978, Unequal visual inputs and strabismus management, a comparison of human and animal strabismus, in: *Symposium on Strabismus. Trans. New Orleans Acad. Ophthalmol.*, Mosby, St. Louis.

Jones, K. R., Spear, P. D., and Tong, L., 1984, Critical periods for effects on monocular deprivation: Differences between striate and extrastriate cortex, *J. Neurosci.* **4**:2543–2552.

Kim, D. S., and Bonhoeffer, T., 1993, Chronic observation of the emergence of iso-orientation domains in kitten visual cortex, *Soc. Neurosci. Abstr.* **19**:1800.

Kiorpes, L., 1989, The development of spatial resolution and contrast sensitivity in naturally strabismic monkeys, *Clin. Vision Sci.* **4**:279–293.

Kiorpes, L., Carlson, M. R., and Alfi, D., 1989, Development of visual acuity in experimentally strabismic monkeys, *Clin. Vision Sci.* **4**:95–106.

LeVay, S., Wiesel, T. N., and Hubel, D. H., 1980, The development of ocular dominance columns in normal and visually deprived monkeys, *J. Comp. Neurol.* **191**:1–51.

Levitt, F. B., and Van Sluyters, R. C., 1982, The sensitive period for strabismus in the kitten, *Dev. Brain Res.* **3**:323–327.

Maurer, D., and Lewis, T. L., 1993, Visual outcomes after infantile cataract, in: *Early Visual Development, Normal and Abnormal* (K. Simons, ed.), Oxford University Press, London, pp. 454–484.

Mitchell, D. E., 1991, The long-term effectiveness of different regimens of occlusion on recovery from early monocular deprivation in kittens, *Philos. Trans. R. Soc. London Ser. B* **333**:51–79.

Mohindra, I., Zwaan, J., Held, R., Brill, S., and Zwaan, F., 1985, Development of acuity and stereopsis in infants with esotropia, *Ophthalmology* **92**:691–697.

Mower, G. D., Caplan, C. J., Christen, W. G., and Duffy, F. H., 1985, Dark rearing prolongs physiological but not anatomical plasticity of the cat visual cortex, *J. Comp. Neurol.* **235**:448–466.

Odom, J. V., Hoyt, C. S., and Marg, E., 1982, Eye patching and visual evoked potential acuity in children four months to eight years old, *Am. J. Optom. Physiol. Opt.* **59**:706–717.

Olson, C. R., and Freeman, R. D., 1980, Profile of the sensitive period for monocular deprivation in kittens, *Exp. Brain Res.* **39**:17–21.

Pettet, M. W., and Gilbert, C. D., 1992, Dynamic changes in receptive-field size in cat primary visual cortex, *Proc. Natl. Acad. Sci. USA* **89**:8366–8370.

Rodman, H. R., 1994, Development of inferior temporal cortex in the monkey, *Cereb. Cortex* **5**:484–498.

Shatz, C. J., and Stryker, M. P., 1978, Ocular dominance in layer IV of the cat's visual cortex and the effects of monocular deprivation, *J. Physiol. (London)* **281**:267–283.

Sherman, S. M., 1985, Development of retinal projections to the cat's lateral geniculate nucleus, *Trends Neurosci.* **8**:350–355.

Sherman, S. M., and Stone, J., 1973, Physiological normality of the retina in visually deprived cats, *Brain Res.* **60**:224–230.

Stryker, M. P., and Harris, W. A., 1986, Binocular impulse blockade prevents the formation of ocular dominance columns in cat visual cortex, *J. Neurosci.* **6**:2117–2133.

Tierney, D. W., 1989, Vision recovery in amblyopia after contralateral subretinal hemorrhage, *J. Am. Optom. Assoc.* **60**:281–283.

Vaegen, and Taylor, D., 1979, Critical period for deprivation amblyopia in children, *Trans. Ophthalmol. Soc. UK* **99**:432–439.

Vereecken, E. P., and Brabant, P., 1984, Prognosis for vision in amblyopia after loss of the good eye, *Arch. Ophthalmol.* **102**:220–224.

von Noorden, G. K., 1990, *Binocular Vision and Ocular Motility*, Mosby, St. Louis.

III

Mechanisms of Plasticity

10

Concepts of Plasticity

The fundamental question that many scientists in the field of visual development are tackling today is: what are the mechanisms that underlie plasticity in the visual cortex? How can the system adapt to abnormalities in the visual environment, and readapt when the abnormality is corrected? How do infants and children have this capability, and why do adults lack it?

In this section, we will discuss mechanisms of sensory-dependent plasticity. There are equally fascinating questions about the initial development of the visual system that depends on molecular cues, which was discussed in Chapter 4. Unfortunately, there is not sufficient space here to go into those questions as well.

In sensory-dependent plasticity, the connections in the visual cortex change in response to an altered sensory input. The change is specific to the input. Ocular dominance is altered by an abnormal balance in the input from the two eyes; orientation selectivity is altered by an emphasis on lines of a particular orientation in the input; direction selectivity is altered by continued motion in one direction, and so on. All of these signals are carried to the cortex by electrical activity; consequently, blockage of activity reaching the cortex with tetrodotoxin prevents sensory-dependent plasticity (see Chapter 4).

The cortical alteration to sensory input is a long-term change in the physiological properties of the cells. In most cases this probably reflects a rearrangement of the anatomical connections. Certainly this is true in monocular deprivation, where the connections between lateral geniculate and cortex are altered. Probably it is also true in orientation changes, in loss of acuity, and in anomalous retinal correspondence, but the currently available anatomical techniques do not permit this point to be tested. The suppression found in strabismus may involve a change in the connections of inhibitory cells, or it may just involve a long-term change in the physiological properties of the synapses. Again, the proof awaits technical advances.

So we can restate the fundamental question: how does a change in the pattern of electrical activity reaching the visual cortex lead to a rearrangement of anatomical connections or long-term changes in the physiological properties of the synapses, and a long-term change in the physiological properties of the cells?

155

There are bound to be a number of steps leading to the anatomical and physiological changes. Electrical activity leads to release of synaptic transmitters, which leads to changes in second messengers within the cell, and changes in protein synthesis for formation of new cell membrane, new cell processes, and new synaptic proteins. So there are really two fundamental questions: (1) What steps lead to the final cortical alterations? (2) Which steps that enable the cortices of young animals to be plastic are absent or reduced in adults?

I. The Hebb Postulate

Many years ago Donald Hebb (1949) proposed that learning takes place by strengthening the transmission at single synapses. He postulated that "when an axon of cell A is near enough to excite cell B and repeatedly or persistently takes part in firing it, some growth process or metabolic change takes place in one or both cells such that A's efficiency, as one of the cells firing B, is increased."

We can expand on this proposition in various respects to take account of current knowledge. First, there must be a weakening of inactive synapses, as well as a strengthening of active ones (Stent, 1973). There has to be forgetting, as well as memory. A single synapse cannot be strengthened indefinitely. The process cannot go in only one direction.

Second, one has to take account of the idea of competition. Active synapses drive out inactive ones, not only in the visual cortex, but also in other systems where the question has been closely studied, such as the neuromuscular junction and various ganglia (Purves and Lichtman, 1980). Hebb's postulate considers what happens at a single synapse, rather than what happens at one synapse compared to others on the same postsynaptic cell.

To illustrate competition, let us consider ocular dominance changes, where the phenomenon of competition is most clearly established. In monocular deprivation, when inputs from the intact eye fire together without inputs from the deprived eye, connections from the deprived eye to the cortex are weakened. With strabismus, inputs from the left and right eyes are not in synchrony, so some cells become totally driven by the left eye, and some totally by the right eye: very few binocular cells are left. The same result occurs if one eye is open, then the other, but both eyes are never open together (Hubel and Wiesel, 1965; Blasdel and Pettigrew, 1979). It also occurs if natural activity is abolished with tetrodotoxin, and the eyes are stimulated electrically out of synchrony with each other (Stryker and Strickland, 1984).

To explain competition, one has to consider that there are several inputs onto the postsynaptic cell, and assume that the postsynaptic cell is only activated if a number of inputs are active at once. In Fig. 10.1, four inputs are shown. One could postulate that the postsynaptic cell only fires when two presynaptic inputs arrive at the same time. Then, the postsynaptic cell will fire in conjunction with the presynaptic input only if two left eye inputs arrive at the same time, two right eye inputs arrive at the same time, or a left eye input and a right eye input arrive at the same time. Synapses that are passive, or only weakly activated, will degenerate. Binocularity will be maintained only if left

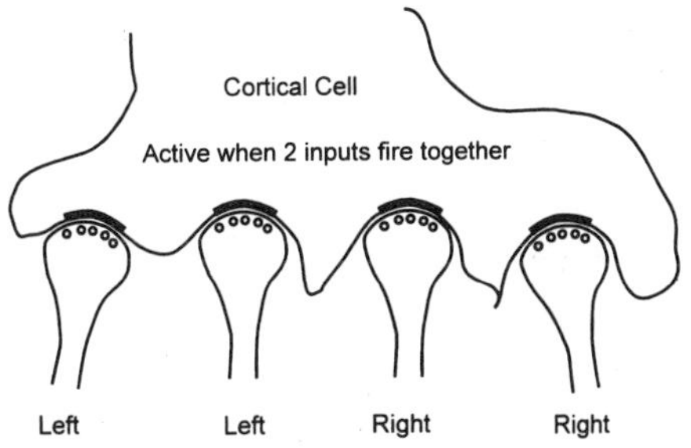

FIG. 10.1. Hebb synapse drawn to take account of competition between left and right eyes in the visual cortex. In this example, the hypothesis is that some process in the postsynaptic cell is activated when two or more inputs arrive together, and will strengthen those synapses that are active and weaken the ones that are not. Reprinted with permission from *Investigative Ophthalmology and Visual Science*, Daw (1994).

and right eye inputs fire together. The left eye will take over if the left eye is active, and the right eye is not. If the two eyes rarely fire in synchrony with each other, then cells initially dominated by the left eye will tend to be taken over by the left eye, and cells initially dominated by the right eye will tend to be taken over by the right eye.

Third, the process that Hebb referred to as "firing" may not be firing of an action potential. The question of what voltage change is required for strengthening of the synapse is important but unresolved. The voltage change leads to entry of calcium into the cell, and it could be that a particular level of calcium in the dendritic spine is important (Zador et al., 1990). The voltage change and/or the calcium change must then trigger a storage process that changes the state of the synapse, so that it becomes potentiated and remains potentiated over a long period of time. The synaptic alteration could be stored by a molecule, such as calcium/calmodulin-dependent kinase (CaM-KII) that has two stable states, and a threshold for conversion from one state to the other (Lisman, 1985). All of these hypotheses are consistent with the Hebb postulate, in the sense that there is in the postsynaptic cell a switch that gets turned on when a sufficient number of presynaptic inputs arrive at the same time.

Fourth, the Hebb synapse model does not consider formation of new synapses, only potentiation of existing synapses. Sprouting of processes almost certainly occurs, and presumably some of these processes form new synapses. So one has to add to the postulate some factor for the generation of these new synapses, which may be random, or could be under the guidance of some molecular cue.

II. How Electrical Activity Can Lead to a Strengthening of Some Synapses and a Weakening of Others

The idea that synapses can be weakened as well as strengthened leads to a problem. The signals are carried to the visual cortex by electrical activity. Electrical activity is always a positive parameter: it can increase from zero, but cannot be negative. One could postulate that there is a certain level of electrical activity above which synapses are strengthened and below which they are weakened (Bienenstock et al., 1982). This could happen if a low level of input were to activate some processes in the postsynaptic cell, and a high level of input were to activate others. However, one has again to take account of the phenomenon of competition, and the point that one cannot account for all of the results on the basis of what happens at a single synapse.

Thus, one has to consider what happens in the postsynaptic cell. Electrical activity will affect a substance or substances in this cell. In one model, the crucial factor is the state of phosphorylation of CaM-KII (Lisman, 1989). All levels of electrical activity lead to entry of calcium into the cell, and to phosphorylation of this molecule. Low levels of calcium activate a calcineurin cascade, leading to dephosphorylation of CaM-KII. High levels of calcium activate cyclic AMP, and turn off the dephosphorylation. Thus, high levels of electrical activity lead to highly phosphorylated CaM-KII, and increase synaptic efficacy, and low levels of electrical activity reduce this. The appealing feature of this model is that it puts clothes onto what are frequently rather bare and theoretical discussions of the problem. However, many issues will have to be resolved before this model, or any other, can be proved. These include the subcellular location of the enzymes, how gradients of calcium within the cell affect the results, and the location of left and right eye inputs in relation to each other and to the enzymes, among others. The main point to be noted at this stage is that the problem is not a simple one.

III. Feedback from the Postsynaptic Cell to the Presynaptic Terminal

The Hebb synapse model requires activation of the postsynaptic cell for the synapse to be strengthened. However, changes also occur in the presynaptic terminals. The best evidence for this comes from monocular deprivation. When one eye is closed, the endings in the visual cortex coming from that eye retract. As pointed out before, this is not simply a degeneration of input from the deprived eye: monocular deprivation, involving competition between active inputs from the normal eye and inactive inputs from the deprived eye, has a much stronger effect on the deprived eye inputs than binocular deprivation, where there is simply inactive input from both eyes. This is evidence that competition for synaptic space on the postsynaptic cell, where binocular convergence occurs, leads to strengthening of some presynaptic terminals, and weakening of others. While the postsynaptic cell must be involved, because there would be no competition without it, the result of the competition is carried back to the presynaptic terminals, and shows up there as a change in the presynaptic terminal arborization.

The point that the postsynaptic cell is involved in electrical effects on synaptic efficacy is reinforced by experiments on orientation-selective deprivation (Rauschecker and Singer, 1979). Kittens were reared in the dark until 5 weeks, then with one eye open for 9 days, then with the other eye open and vertical lines blurred by a strong cylindrical lens over that eye for another 10 days. Only the postsynaptic cells in the visual cortex are specific for orientation. During the reverse suture, the cells in the visual cortex specific for horizontal lines will be driven through the reopened eye, but the cells specific for vertical lines will not. Thus, if the postsynaptic cell is involved, one would expect ocular dominance to be reversed by the second exposure for horizontal lines but not for vertical ones. This is what occurred. The final result in the case of ocular dominance changes is alterations in the presynaptic terminals, in that they are known to retract from the postsynaptic cell. This experiment therefore also suggests that there is a feedback signal from the postsynaptic cell to the presynaptic terminals.

Thus, the Hebb model, with modifications, fits the general results obtained in the visual cortex from sensory deprivation. When pre- and postsynaptic cells are activated together, the synapse between them is strengthened. When they are not activated together, the synapse is weakened. The postsynaptic cell is not activated unless several presynaptic inputs arrive at the same time. Consequently, the pattern of presynaptic inputs is important. The presynaptic inputs compete with each other for space on the postsynaptic cell. The final result is not only a change in synaptic efficacy, but also a change in the terminal arbor of the presynaptic cell, implying a feedback signal from the postsynaptic cell to the presynaptic terminal.

IV. Criteria for Critical Factors in the Critical Period

This discussion of the Hebb synapse shows that there must be a series of processes and reactions involved between the electrical activity that guides plastic changes in the visual cortex, and the axonal and dendritic alterations that eventually result. The electrical activity leads to release of the synaptic transmitter glutamate, activation of glutamate receptors, activation of second messengers, various reactions within the postsynaptic cell, and the feedback signal from the postsynaptic cell to the presynaptic terminals. In nearly all cases the model has been monocular deprivation (Fig. 10.2). A number of factors and substances have been shown to affect these processes.

In determining whether or not a factor is actually important in plasticity, the first test is usually to see if removal of the factor, or application of an antagonist, reduces or abolishes plasticity. In the monocular deprivation model, this means: Are the ocular dominance changes that normally occur after monocular deprivation disrupted? Such experiments lead to a long list of putative factors (Table 10.1). Some items on the list definitely represent important

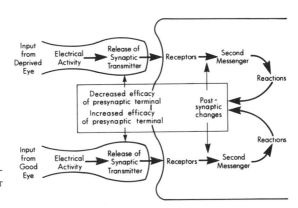

FIG. 10.2. Steps involved in plasticity in the visual cortex, using ocular dominance changes as a model.

TABLE 10.1. Some Factors and Substances That Reduce or Abolish Ocular Dominance Shifts in Cat Visual Cortex

- Tetrodotoxin (Stryker and Harris, 1986)
- Infusion of antagonists to the NMDA receptor (Kleinschmidt *et al.*, 1987)
- Reduction of noradrenaline and acetylcholine input to the cortex (Bear and Singer, 1986)
- Injection of cortisol (Daw *et al.*, 1991)
- Infusion of nerve growth factor (Carmignoto *et al.*, 1993)
- Lesions of the internal medullary lamina and medial dorsal nucleus in the thalamus (Singer, 1982)
- Infusion of glutamate into the cortex (Shaw and Cynader, 1984)
- Anesthesia and paralysis (Freeman and Bonds, 1979)

contributors to the regulation of plasticity. The prime example of this has already been discussed: tetrodotoxin, which abolishes electrical activity, also abolishes plasticity in the visual cortex because the signals that guide plasticity are carried by the neurons in the visual pathway.

Other items on the list influence plasticity, but do not contribute directly to it. One example is reduction of the noradrenaline and acetylcholine input to the cortex (Bear and Singer, 1986). The afferents that use these transmitters come from the brain stem, and carry signals about the sleep/wake cycle and the general state of attention. Interruption of both of these pathways with a combination of lesions and antagonists affects ocular dominance changes. Exactly how this might occur is unknown, but probably acetylcholine and noradrenaline affect the state of depolarization and/or second messengers of the cells in the visual pathway, and thereby accentuate or reduce the signals in those pathways. In another example, lesions of the intermedullary lamina and medial dorsal nucleus of the thalamus reduce ocular dominance changes (Singer, 1982). These are areas that also have to do with attention, and with eye movements. It has not yet been determined whether it is the effect of the lesions on attention, or the effect on eye movements that is crucial, but in either case, the influence is one that affects the visual pathway, rather than one that is on the visual pathway. To emphasize the point, Singer describes such results as "gating" control of plasticity. The signals are not on the pathway for sensory-dependent control of connections in the visual cortex, but they may gate those signals.

Other items on the list have general nonspecific actions on the nervous system, and affect all aspects of activity there. One example is anesthesia and paralysis (Freeman and Bonds, 1979): since anesthesia is a general depressant of activity in all parts of the nervous system, it is no surprise that it abolishes plasticity. Another example is infusion of glutamate directly into the cortex (Shaw and Cynader, 1984). Glutamate excites all cells in the nervous system, to such an extent that it can kill them. This is another general nonspecific action. Consequently, the fact that a factor or substance reduces or abolishes plasticity is suggestive, but certainly not conclusive, that it is directly involved in plasticity. Other pieces of supporting evidence must also be assembled.

The complete series of reactions that are directly involved in plasticity will involve some, such as electrical activity, that are there at all ages, and others that are more abundant or more active in the young animal than in the adult.

The latter can be said to be crucial or critical for plasticity, because it is their presence in the young animal that makes the young animal more plastic. Factors or substances that are crucial for plasticity should have a time course of expression that follows the critical period for plasticity. Moreover, this time course should vary with cortical layer, just as the critical period varies with layer. The factor or substance should disappear from layer IV earlier than it disappears from layers II, III, V, and VI.

As an example, consider the class of glutamate receptors called NMDA receptors. The total number of NMDA receptors in the visual cortex follows the critical period quite closely (Gordon *et al.*, 1991; see Fig. 10.3). As a counterexample, the growth-associated protein GAP-43 is associated with plasticity in the hippocampus (Lovinger *et al.*, 1985), and is therefore a candidate to be involved in plasticity in the visual cortex. However, this protein has a concentration that is high shortly after birth in cat visual cortex, and declines to values that are close to adult at the peak of the critical period (McIntosh *et al.*, 1990; see Fig. 10.4). The protein is also associated with growth cones (Skene *et al.*, 1986), suggesting another function: the time during which it is high is when axons are finding their way to their targets, rather than after they have formed synapses, and the synapses are being modified in response to sensory input. Both of these substances are clearly involved in development, but the time course of their change with age suggests that NMDA receptors may be critically involved in sensory-dependent plasticity, whereas GAP-43 is primarily involved in events that occur before sensory-dependent plasticity.

The one treatment that can vary the time course of the critical period is to rear animals in the dark. This causes the critical period to last longer (Cynader and Mitchell, 1980), and delays its onset as well (Mower, 1991). Thus, at 5–6 weeks of age, light-reared animals are more plastic than dark-reared; at 8–9 weeks of age, they are equally plastic; and at 12–20 weeks of age, dark-reared animals are more plastic than light-reared. If a factor or substance is critically involved in plasticity, its concentration should vary similarly between light- and dark-reared animals.

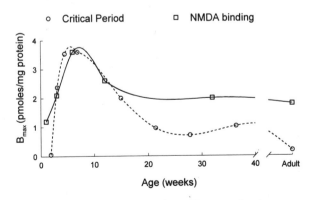

FIG. 10.3. B_{max} for binding of MK801 to NMDA channels in cat visual cortex as a function of age, compared to the critical period for ocular dominance plasticity. Curve for the critical period taken from Fig. 9.1, and scaled to be the same height as B_{max} for MK801 binding at the peak. Reprinted with permission from *Investigative Ophthalmology and Visual Science*, Daw (1994).

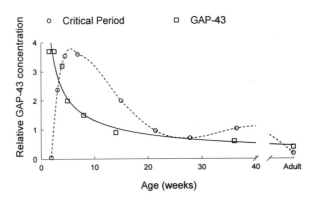

FIG. 10.4. Levels of GAP-43 in the cat visual cortex, compared to the critical period for ocular dominance plasticity. Reprinted with permission from *Investigative Ophthalmology and Visual Science*, Daw (1994).

Finally, a substance that is critically involved in plasticity might bring back plasticity in adult animals. However, there are several caveats to this possibility. First, there may be more than one critical factor in plasticity. If so, then introducing one of them into the adult without also introducing the others may not help. Second, there may be an irreversible process of development, which depends on the critical factors, and which, when set into place, becomes set forever. At one time, some authors thought that the critical period for ocular dominance was directly related to the period over which the geniculocortical afferents segregate in layer IV and that the critical period in layer IV might come to an end when this segregation had taken place. Now most authors believe that the critical period for ocular dominance shifts lasts longer than the period of ocular dominance segregation: shifts in ocular dominance can occur after the period of segregation in normal animals is over (LeVay *et al.*, 1980; Swindale *et al.*,, 1981). However, the concept that there is an irreversible step has to be considered.

The possibility that plasticity could be brought back after the critical period has almost never been tested, at least partly because of these caveats. It may not be possible to test it adequately until the complete series of reactions that is directly involved in plasticity has been defined. Nevertheless this is the possibility that most people in the field are working toward. The hope is that, several years down the road, after the whole process is understood, it will be practical to bring back plasticity in older animals.

V. Summary

Electrical activity in the afferents to the visual cortex leads to a series of reactions in cells in the cortex. These reactions affect the strength of the synapses between the presynaptic terminals and the postsynaptic cell. Active synapses are strengthened, and inactive ones are weakened. A combination of inputs may be required to drive the reactions in the postsynaptic cell, so that inputs that are activated together will strengthen each other, and inputs that are not activated together will be weakened. The series of reactions includes feed-back to the presynaptic terminals, and morphological changes there. Some of the steps in the series of reactions will be found in the cortex at all ages. Others will be found at a higher level, or with higher activity, at the peak of the critical period for plasticity. The latter are the steps that are critical for plasticity.

We can define three criteria for a factor or substance that is critical for plasticity:

1. Removing the factor, or providing antagonists to the substance, should reduce or abolish plasticity.
2. The presence or activity of the factor or substance should follow the time course of the critical period for plasticity.
3. Treatments that affect the critical period for plasticity should affect the factor or substance similarly.

In addition, it is possible that reintroducing the critical factors or substances after the critical period is over may bring plasticity back again. After all of the steps directly involved in plasticity have been defined, this criterion will also need to be fulfilled.

Various factors and substances that could be involved in plasticity will be discussed and evaluated by these criteria in Chapter 12 after the phenomenon of long-term potentiation has been described.

References

Bear, M. F., and Singer, W., 1986, Modulation of visual cortical plasticity by acetylcholine and noradrenaline, *Nature* **320**:172–176.

Bienenstock, E. L., Cooper, L. N., and Munro, P. W., 1982, Theory for the development of neuron selectivity: Orientation specificity and binocular interaction in visual cortex, *J. Neurosci.* **2**:32–48.

Blasdel, G. G., and Pettigrew, J. D., 1979, Degree of interocular synchrony required for maintenance of binocularity in kitten's visual cortex, *J. Neurophysiol.* **42**:1692–1710.

Carmignoto, G., Canella, R., Candeo, P., Comelli, M. C., and Maffei, L., 1993, Effects of nerve growth factor on neuronal plasticity of the kitten visual cortex, *J. Physiol. (London)* **464**:343–360.

Cynader, M. S., and Mitchell, D. E., 1980, Prolonged sensitivity to monocular deprivation in dark-reared cats, *J. Neurophysiol.* **43**:1026–1040.

Daw, N. W., 1994, Mechanisms of plasticity in the visual cortex, *Invest. Ophthalmol. Vis. Sci.* **35**:4168–4179.

Daw, N. W., Sato, H., Fox, K., Carmichael, T., and Gingerich, R., 1991, Cortisol reduces plasticity in the kitten visual cortex, *J. Neurobiol.* **22**:158–168.

Freeman, R. D., and Bonds, A. B., 1979, Cortical plasticity in monocularly deprived immobilized kittens depends on eye movement, *Science* **206**:1093–1095.

Gordon, B., Daw, N. W., and Parkinson, D., 1991, The effect of age on binding of MK-801 in the cat visual cortex, *Dev. Brain Res.* **62**:61–68.

Hebb, D. O., 1949, *The Organization of Behaviour*, Wiley, New York, p. 62.

Hubel, D. H., and Wiesel, T. N., 1965, Binocular interaction in striate cortex of kittens reared with artificial squint, *J. Neurophysiol.* **28**:1041–1059.

Kleinschmidt, A., Bear, M. F., and Singer, W., 1987, Blockade of "NMDA" receptors disrupts experience-dependent plasticity of kitten striate cortex, *Science* **238**:355–358.

LeVay, S., Wiesel, T. N., and Hubel, D. H., 1980, The development of ocular dominance columns in normal and visually deprived monkeys, *J. Comp. Neurol.* **191**:1–51.

Lisman, J. E., 1985, A mechanism for memory storage insensitive to molecular turnover: A bistable autophosphorylating kinase, *Proc. Natl. Acad. Sci. USA* **82**:3055–3057.

Lisman, J., 1989, A mechanism for the Hebb and the anti-Hebb processes underlying learning and memory *Proc. Natl. Acad. Sci. USA* **86**:9574–9578.

Lovinger, D. M., Akers, R. F., Nelson, R. B., Barnes, C. A., McNaughton, B. L., and Routtenberg, A., 1985, A selective increase in phosphorylation of protein F1, a protein kinase C substrate, directly related to three day growth of long term synaptic enhancement, *Brain Res.* **343**:137–143.

McIntosh, H., Daw, N. W., and Parkinson, D., 1990, GAP-43 in the cat visual cortex during postnatal development, *Vis. Neurosci.* **4**:585–594.

Mower, G. D., 1991, The effect of dark rearing on the time course of the critical period in cat visual cortex, *Dev. Brain Res.* **58**:151–158.

Purves, D., and Lichtman, J. W., 1980, Elimination of synapses in the developing nervous system, *Science* **210**:153–157.

Rauschecker, J. P., and Singer, W., 1979, Changes in the circuitry of the kitten visual cortex are gated by postsynaptic activity, *Nature* **280**:58–60.

Shaw, C., and Cynader, M. S., 1984, Disruption of cortical activity prevents ocular dominance changes in monocularly deprived kittens, *Nature* **308**:731–734.

Singer, W., 1982, Central core control of developmental plasticity in the kitten visual cortex: I. Diencephalic lesions, *Exp. Brain Res.* **47**:209–222.

Skene, J. H. P., Jacobson, R. D., Snipes, G. J., McGuire, C. B., Norden, J. J., and Freeman, J. A., 1986, A protein induced during nerve growth (GAP43) is a major component of growth-cone membranes, *Science* **233**:783–786.

Stent, G. S., 1973, A physiological mechanism for Hebb's postulate of learning, *Proc. Natl. Acad. Sci. USA* **70**:997–1001.

Stryker, M. P., and Harris, W. A., 1986, Binocular impulse blockade prevents the formation of ocular dominance columns in cat visual cortex, *J. Neurosci.* **6**:2117–2133.

Stryker, M. P., and Strickland, S. L., 1984, Physiological segregation of ocular dominance columns depends on the pattern of afferent electrical activity, *Invest. Ophthalmol. Suppl.* **25**:278.

Swindale, N. V., Vital-Durand, F., and Blakemore, C., 1981, Recovery from monocular deprivation in the monkey. III. Reversal of anatomical effects in the visual cortex, *Proc. R. Soc. Lond B. Biol. Sci.* **213**:435–450.

Zador, A., Koch, C., and Brown, T. H., 1990, Biophysical model of a Hebbian synapse, *Proc. Natl. Acad. Sci. USA* **87**:6718–6722.

11

Long-Term Potentiation as a Model

Long-term potentiation (LTP) is a strengthening of synaptic transmission that was first discovered in the hippocampus (Bliss and Lomo, 1973). If one stimulates the afferents to the hippocampus at a high rate (100 Hz for 3 sec), the excitatory postsynaptic potentials in the hippocampal pyramidal cells are subsequently found to be larger than normal, and to rise more quickly. The effect lasts for several hours, and can last for as long as the preparation does.

An enormous amount has been learned about LTP in the last 10 years. Experiments can be done on slices in a dish, where a number of manipulations can be performed. Consequently, progress is much more rapid than with sensory-dependent plasticity in the visual cortex, where each experiment takes days to weeks rather than hours. Moreover, there is long-term depression as well as LTP, triggered by stimulation at a low rate (1 Hz for 15 min; Dudek and Bear, 1992).

LTP is found in the visual cortex as well as the hippocampus (Tsumoto and Suda, 1979; Komatsu et al., 1988). It could underlie sensory-dependent plasticity, but there are several differences between the two phenomena. First, LTP is found in layers II and III of adult visual cortex, after the critical period for sensory-dependent plasticity is over (Artola and Singer, 1987). Second, the time course of LTP and sensory-dependent plasticity are very different. LTP occurs after a single burst of stimuli, whereas sensory-dependent plasticity takes hours or days of stimulation before results are seen. Third, LTP is primarily a physiological phenomenon. It may lead to some morphological changes (see Lisman and Harris, 1993), but expansion and retraction of presynaptic terminals like those seen after monocular deprivation have not been clearly demonstrated.

Nevertheless, LTP could be an early step in the series of reactions involved in sensory-dependent plasticity. Unfortunately, no one has yet devised an experiment to prove this. Moreover, it is not clear that such an experiment is possible (I have an offer open for a dinner at the most expensive restaurant in either New Haven or New York, for anyone who proposes such an experiment, because it would save me a large amount of time; so far, no one has tried to collect!). Until such an experiment is done, we have to take results from LTP as a guide to some of the steps that could be involved in sensory-dependent plasticity, then use the visual cortex to prove that they actually are involved in sensory-dependent plasticity. The power of LTP is that results come in rapidly, and yield lots of clues to be tested by the slower methods available for studying sensory-dependent plasticity in whole animals.

I. Steps Involved in Long-Term Potentiation

LTP is triggered, like sensory-dependent plasticity, by electrical activity. The transmitter that is released by electrical activity in the visual cortex is glutamate. Glutamate acts on three classes of receptor in the postsynaptic cell (Fig. 11.1). The first is called AMPA/kainate, after the agonists α-amino-3-hydroxy-5-methyl-isoxazole-4-propionate (AMPA) and kainate, which are specific for different receptors in the class. AMPA/kainate receptors open channels that let cations into the cell. The second class is called NMDA receptors, after the specific agonist N-methyl-D-aspartate. The NMDA receptor also lets cations (calcium as well as sodium) into the cell. The third class is called metabotropic, because receptors in this class act on G-proteins, which in turn act on second messengers such as cyclic AMP or phosphoinositides, but do not directly open channels. There are at least six types of receptor in each of these classes (see Nakanishi, 1992).

All three classes of glutamate receptor contribute to LTP, although not all are required for it. LTP does not occur in the presence of the NMDA antagonist D-amino-phosphonovalerate (APV) (Collingridge et al., 1983). LTP also does not occur in the presence of the metabotropic antagonist RS-α-methyl-4-carboxyphenylglycine (MCPG) (Bashir et al., 1993), although this result is still controversial. LTP does occur in the presence of an antagonist specific for the AMPA/kainate receptors (Kauer et al., 1988; Muller et al., 1988), but AMPA/kainate receptors probably contribute to LTP by depolarizing the neuron, and activating NMDA receptors. Very likely more than one glutamate receptor has to be activated, because stimulation of the input with NMDA does not, by itself, lead to LTP (Collingridge et al., 1983), but LTP can be produced by perfusion with NMDA and the metabotropic glutamate agonist 1-aminocyclopentane-trans-1,3-dicarboxylic acid (ACPD) at the same time (Musgrave et al., 1993).

There has been particular interest in the role of the NMDA receptor in LTP. This is because the NMDA receptor channel is voltage sensitive. Near resting potential for the cell, at -70 mV, the current flowing through the NMDA chan-

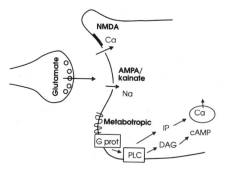

FIG. 11.1. The three types of glutamate receptor. AMPA/kainate receptors open ion channels that let sodium into the cell. The NMDA receptor is connected to an ion channel that lets calcium into the cell as well as sodium. Metabotropic receptors are connected to G proteins which activate phospholipase C (PLC), which produces inositol phosphate (IP) and diacylglycerol (DAG). Inositol phosphate releases calcium from intracellular stores. Diacylglycerol affects the concentration of cyclic AMP.

nel is reduced, because the channel is partially blocked by magnesium ions. When the cell is depolarized, the channel becomes unblocked, and the current flowing through the channel increases, to a peak at -30 mV. In other words, the NMDA channel is turned on at high levels of activity. There is a substantial contribution from NMDA receptors to the response in the hippocampus when afferents are stimulated at 100 Hz, but not when they are stimulated at less than 10 Hz (Collingridge *et al.*, 1988).

At one time, it was thought that the NMDA channel might act as a switch, because of its voltage-sensitive properties. If it did act as a switch, then this might be the crucial step that turns on LTP at high levels of activity. However, this does not appear to be the case, at least in the visual cortex of the intact animal (Fox *et al.*, 1990). Activation of the NMDA receptor does not produce a result like the action potential, where the membrane potential changes in a rapid all-or-nothing fashion. As the concentration of NMDA is increased, the response in the postsynaptic cell is a graded change (Fox and Daw, 1992). What the NMDA receptor does do is to amplify the incoming signals, and steepen the input/output curve across the synapse.

The NMDA receptor also lets calcium into the cell (Dingledine, 1983). This is an important step in the activation of LTP. Chelation of calcium in the postsynaptic cell with EGTA blocks the induction of LTP (Lynch *et al.*, 1983), and an increase in the level of calcium in the postsynaptic cell potentiates synaptic transmission (Malenka *et al.*, 1988). There are actually two other sources of calcium, besides the calcium that flows in through NMDA channels. One is voltage-sensitive calcium channels in the cell membrane, which are activated by depolarization of the neuron. The other source is intracellular calcium stores, which are activated to release calcium by phosphoinositides, which in turn are activated by metabotropic glutamate receptors. Substantial amounts of calcium can enter the cell through the voltage-gated calcium channels (Miyakawa *et al.*, 1992), although entry of calcium through these channels alone does not trigger LTP (Malenka *et al.*, 1989b). Blockade of release of calcium from the intracellular stores can block the induction of LTP (Obenaus *et al.*, 1989; Alford *et al.*, 1993). Consequently, release of calcium from all three sources may play some role in the process.

Indeed, calcium may be a more important contributor to LTP, as a general rule, than NMDA receptors. In some parts of the hippocampus, LTP may be activated by increases in calcium, without the participation of NMDA receptors (Zalutsky and Nicoll, 1990). The same phenomenon can be seen in the visual cortex (Komatsu and Iwakiri, 1992). While NMDA receptors are generally activated, and calcium entry through NMDA receptors is a crucial component leading to LTP, an increase in calcium coming from other sources may also lead to LTP.

Calcium activates the enzyme calmodulin, and calmodulin in turn activates calcium/calmodulin-dependent protein kinase II (CaM-KII), which is a major component of postsynaptic densities. Specific inhibitors of CaM-KII block LTP (Malenka *et al.*, 1989a; Malinow *et al.*, 1989). Moreover, LTP is affected in mice that have been genetically altered, so that they do not produce the α form of CaM-KII (Silva *et al.*, 1992). It seems likely, therefore, that CaM-KII plays some role in LTP.

The enzyme protein kinase C (PKC) has also been implicated in LTP. PKC can be activated by diacylglycerol through metabotropic glutamate receptors, G-proteins, and phospholipase C; some forms of PKC can also be activated by calcium. Consequently, both NMDA and metabotropic glutamate receptors may play a role in the activation of PKC. There is increased activity of PKC during the maintenance of LTP (Klann et al., 1991). Activation of PKC can prolong LTP (Lovinger and Routtenberg, 1988). Moreover, inhibition of PKC in the post-synaptic cell by injection of inhibitors directly into that cell blocks LTP (Malenka et al., 1989a; Malinow et al., 1989). The conclusion is that PKC is an essential step along the pathway for LTP.

Numerous other enzymes may play a role in LTP. PKC and CaM-KII are both serine-threonine kinases. Some form of tyrosine kinase is also involved, since broad-spectrum tyrosine kinase inhibitors that do not affect serine-threonine kinases also interfere with LTP (O'Dell et al., 1991b). However, exactly where and how these inhibitors act in the chain of reactions has not been determined. Activation of NMDA receptors by high frequencies of stimulation also leads to an increase in cAMP (Chetkovitch et al., 1991), which is probably involved in the later phases of LTP (Frey et al., 1993).

One has to consider the mechanism for long-term depression (LTD) as well as LTP. Both are elicited by stimulation. LTP is produced by a burst at 100 Hz, and LTD by stimulation at 1 Hz. Indeed, one can produce LTP by high-frequency stimulation, and then abolish it by low-frequency stimulation—a phenomenon known as depotentiation. LTD also involves NMDA receptors and influx of calcium, just as LTP does (Dudek and Bear, 1992; Mulkey and Malenka, 1992). The current theory is that the sequence of reactions involved in LTP and LTD is the same for the first four steps: electrical activity leads to release of glutamate, activation of glutamate receptors, and changes of calcium levels in the cell, although the source of the calcium may differ in the two situations (Kato, 1993). Indeed, the same stimulus can produce LTP or LTD, depending on the level of calcium in the cell (Mulkey and Malenka, 1992). Thereafter the reactions are thought to be different: high levels of calcium activate some enzymes to produce LTP and low levels of calcium activate others to produce LTD (Lisman, 1989).

Currently, the amount of work done on LTD is much less than that done on LTP. There is evidence that LTD produced by low-frequency stimulation can be blocked by protein phosphatase inhibitors (Mulkey et al., 1993) and calcineurin inhibitors (Mulkey et al., 1994). These results support the theory mentioned above (Lisman, 1989), but other reactions have to be involved. Clearly, considerably more work needs to be done before the mechanisms are worked out.

In the long run, LTP must involve protein synthesis. The synaptic changes could not occur without some form of protein synthesis. In intact animals, protein synthesis inhibitors block LTP (Stanton and Sarvey, 1984), and the inhibitor anisomycin specifically blocks later phases rather than the initial ones (Krug et al., 1984). There is also a period in which protein synthesis can occur from existing messenger RNA, followed by a period in which new mRNA must be made (Otani et al., 1989). Presumably a wide variety of proteins need to be made, with different proteins involved in different aspects of the physiological and anatomical changes that occur. Some have been studied; for example, the protein MAP-2, which is a dendrite component, is dephosphorylated by activation of NMDA receptors (Halpain and Greengard, 1990). The full list of required proteins will probably turn out to be quite predictable, since it must draw on the list of proteins known to be involved in cell membranes and the various aspects of synaptic transmission. However, the list remains to be worked out.

II. Feedback Factors

With LTP, as with sensory-dependent plasticity, there is good evidence that the mechanism includes feedback to the presynaptic terminal. The postsynaptic cell must be activated for LTP to be established, as described above. However, there are also effects on the presynaptic cell that lead to long-term changes in it. In particular, LTP leads to an increased concentration of glutamate found in the extracellular space, coming from the presynaptic terminals (Bliss et al., 1990).

Two candidates have emerged for the molecule that carries the signal from the postsynaptic cell back to the presynaptic cell. One is arachidonic acid, a fatty acid. The other is nitric oxide, a gas. There may also be structural changes in the synapse itself that involve both pre- and postsynaptic membranes (Lisman and Harris, 1993).

A number of experiments have been done to study the relationship of arachidonic acid to LTP. LTP leads to an increase in the concentration of arachidonic acid in extracellular space (Bliss et al., 1990). This release can be activated by NMDA receptors (Dumuis et al., 1988). Inhibition of the production of arachidonic acid blocks the induction of LTP (Lynch et al., 1989). Moreover, perfusion with arachidonic acid, accompanied by weak activation, produces a slow and persistent increase in synaptic efficacy in the hippocampus (Williams et al., 1989). Arachidonic acid may stimulate transmitter release by stimulating phosphoinositide turnover (Bliss et al., 1990), or it may prolong the effect of glutamate on the postsynaptic cell by inhibiting uptake of glutamate (Barbour et al., 1989). These various pieces of evidence suggest that arachidonic acid may be a retrograde transmitter for later phases of LTP, but more experiments are needed to clarify the details.

Nitric oxide (NO) is produced in the conversion of arginine to citrulline by nitric oxide synthase. It diffuses readily across synaptic membranes. It activates guanylate cyclase to produce cyclic GMP and also ADP-ribosyl-transferase. For it to be a retrograde messenger, therefore, there has to be NO synthase in the postsynaptic cell; guanylate cyclase or ADP-ribosyl-transferase in the presynaptic cell should affect transmitter release; NO synthase inhibitors should prevent LTP; and production of NO should produce LTP. The evidence on all of these points is controversial. While four groups have reported that NO synthase inhibitors prevent LTP and some that NO donors produce LTP (Bohme et al., 1991; O'Dell et al., 1991a; Schuman and Madison, 1991; Haley et al., 1992), these results have not been replicated by other groups (see Bliss and Collingridge, 1993). The effect of NO synthase inhibitors on LTP varies with temperature, and the strength of the tetanus used to produce the LTP (Williams et al., 1993; Gribkoff and Lum-Ragan, 1992; Haley *et al.*, 1993). Moreover, NO synthase inhibitors have little effect on spatial learning and LTP *in vivo* (Bannerman *et al.*, 1994a,b). Much more work therefore needs to be done before NO is established as a retrograde transmitter.

III. Summary

A series of steps in the pathway leading to LTP and LTD have been worked out (Fig. 11.2). Electrical activity leads to release of glutamate, which activates three classes of glutamate receptor—AMPA/kainate, NMDA, and metabotropic. NMDA receptors play a particular role, because they are turned on more strongly at the high frequencies of stimulation that lead to LTP, and they are involved in both LTP and LTD. NMDA receptors let calcium into the cell, and calcium influx leads to both LTP and LTD. Metabotropic glutamate receptors activate cAMP and also phosphoinositides, which release calcium from internal stores.

The pathways for LTP and LTD are probably identical up to the increase in calcium that can occur from stimulation of all three classes of glutamate receptor. After that they diverge. There is some evidence that the serine-threonine kinases, PKC and calcium/calmodulin-dependent kinase, are involved in LTP, and some tyrosine kinases may be important as well. Phosphatases and calcineurin may be involved in LTD.

There has to be a factor that feeds signals back from the postsynaptic cell to the presynaptic cell. LTP does not occur if various reactions are blocked in the postsynaptic cell, but some of the changes that maintain LTP, such as an increased release of glutamate, must involve changes in the presynaptic cell. There are currently two candidates for the feedback factor: arachidonic acid and nitric oxide. The evidence is not yet conclusive about either of them.

In the final analysis, synthesis of a wide variety of proteins must be involved for the anatomical changes that result from LTP, and probably also for some of the physiological changes. An important consideration in understanding LTP is the localization within the cell of the various proteins and chemical reactions that lead to LTP. A lot of processing probably takes place within the

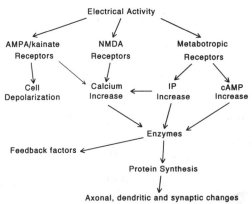

FIG. 11.2. Steps in the pathway for LTP.

dendritic spine. How the enzymes are localized within dendritic spines, within dendrites, and within other parts of the cell remains to be worked out.

All of this represents a remarkable amount of work completed over the last 10 years, and provides some clear pointers for steps that may be involved in plasticity in the visual cortex. Which ones actually are involved will be discussed in the next chapter.

References

Alford, S., Frenguelli, B. G., Schofield, J. G., and Collingridge, G. L., 1993, Characterization of Ca^{2+} signals induced in hippocampal CA1 neurones by the synaptic activation of NMDA receptors, *J. Physiol. (London)* **469**:693–716.

Artola, A., and Singer, W., 1987, Long-term potentiation and NMDA receptors in rat visual cortex, *Nature* **330**:649–652.

Bannerman, D. M., Chapman, P. F., Kelly, P. A. T., Butcher, S. P., and Morris, R. G. M., 1994a, Inhibition of nitric oxide synthase does not impair spatial learning, *J. Neurosci.* **14**:7404–7414.

Bannerman, D. M., Chapman, P. F., Kelly, P. A. T., Butcher, S. P., and Morris, R. G. M., 1994b, Inhibition of nitric oxide synthase does not prevent the induction of long-term potentiation in vivo, *J. Neurosci.* **14**:7415–7425.

Barbour, B., Szatkowski, M., Ingledew, N., and Attwell, D., 1989, Arachidonic acid induces a prolonged inhibition of glutamate uptake into glial cells, *Nature* **342**:918–920.

Bashir, Z. I., Bortolotto, Z. A., Davies, C. H., Beretta, N., Irving, A. J., Seal, A. J., Henley, J. M., Jane, D. E., Watkins, J. C., and Collingridge, G. L., 1993, Induction of LTP in the hippocampus needs synaptic activation of glutamate metabotropic receptors, *Nature* **363**:347–350.

Bliss, T. V. P., and Collingridge, G. L., 1993, A synaptic model of memory: Long-term potentiation in the hippocampus, *Nature* **361**:31–39.

Bliss, T. V. P., and Lomo, T., 1973, Long-lasting potentiation of synaptic transmission in the dentate area of the anesthetized rabbit following stimulation of the perforant path, *J. Physiol. (London)* **232**:331–356.

Bliss, T. V. P., Errington, M. L., Lynch, M. A., and Williams, J. H., 1990, Presynaptic mechanisms in hippocampal long-term potentiation, *Cold Spring Harbor Symp. Quant. Biol.* **55**:119–129.

Bohme, G. A., Bon, C., Stutzmann, J. M., Doble, A., and Blanchard, J. C., 1991, Possible involvement of nitric oxide in long-term potentiation, *Eur. J. Pharmacol.* **199**:379–381.

Chetkovitch, D. M., Gray, R., Johnston, D., and Sweatt, J. D., 1991, N-methyl-D-aspartate receptor activation increases cAMP levels and voltage-gated Ca^{2+} channel activity in area CA1 of hippocampus, *Proc. Natl. Acad. Sci. USA* **88**:6467–6471.

Collingridge, G. L., Kehl, S. J., and McLennan, H., 1983, Excitatory amino acids in synaptic transmission in the Schaffer collateral-commissural pathway of the rat hippocampus, *J. Physiol. (London)* **334**:33–46.

Collingridge, G. L., Herron, C. E., and Lester, R. A. J., 1988, Frequency-dependent N-methyl-D-aspartate receptor-mediated synaptic transmission in rat hippocampus, *J. Physiol. (London)* **399**:301–312.

Dingledine, R., 1983, N-methyl aspartate activates voltage-dependent calcium conductance in rat hippocampal pyramidal cells, *J. Physiol. (London)* **343**:385–405.

Dudek, S. M., and Bear, M. F., 1992, Homosynaptic long-term depression in area CA1 of hippocampus and effects of N-methyl-D-aspartate receptor blockade, *Proc. Natl. Acad. Sci. USA* **89**:4363–4367.

Dumuis, A., Sebben, M., Haynes, L., Pin, J. P., and Bockaert, J., 1988, NMDA receptors activate the arachidonic acid cascade system in striatal neurons, *Nature* **336**:68–70.

Fox, K., and Daw, N. W., 1992, A model for the action of NMDA conductances in the visual cortex, *Neural Computation* **4**:59–83.

Fox, K., Sato, H., and Daw, N. W., 1990, The effect of varying stimulus intensity on NMDA-receptor activity in cat visual cortex, *J. Neurophysiol.* **64**:1413–1428.

Frey, U., Huang, Y. Y., and Kandel, E. R., 1993, Effects of cAMP simulate a late stage of LTP in hippocampal CA1 neurons, *Science* **260**:1661–1664.

Gribkoff, V. K., and Lum-Ragan, J. T., 1992, Evidence for nitric oxide synthase inhibitor-sensitive and insensitive hippocampal synaptic potentiation, *J. Neurophysiol.* **68**:639–642.

Haley, J. E., Wilcox, G. L., and Chapman, P. F., 1992, The role of nitric oxide in hippocampal long-term potentiation, *Neuron* **8**:211–216.

Haley, J. E., Malen, P. L., and Chapman, P. F., 1993, Nitric oxide synthase inhibitors block LTP induced by weak but not strong tetanic stimulation, *Soc. Neurosci. Abstr.* **19**:906.

Halpain, S., and Greengard, P., 1990, Activation of NMDA receptors induces rapid dephosphorylation of the cytoskeletal protein MAP2, *Neuron* **5**:237–246.

Kato, N., 1993, Dependence of long-term depression on postsynaptic metabotropic glutamate receptors in visual cortex, *Proc. Natl. Acad. Sci. USA* **90**:3650–3654.

Kauer, J. A., Malenka, R. C., and Nicoll, R. A., 1988, A persistent postsynaptic modification mediates long-term potentiation in the hippocampus, *Neuron* **1**:911–917.

Klann, E., Chen, S. J., and Sweatt, J. D., 1991, Persistent protein kinase activation in the maintenance phase of long-term potentiation, *J. Biol. Chem.* **266**:24253–24256.

Komatsu, Y., and Iwakiri, M., 1992, Low-threshold Ca^{2+} channels mediate induction of long-term potentiation in kitten visual cortex, *J. Neurophysiol.* **67**:401–410.

Komatsu, Y., Fujii, K., Maeda, J., Sakaguchi, H., and Toyama, K., 1988, Long-term potentiation of synaptic transmission in kitten visual cortex, *J. Neurophysiol.* **59**:124–141.

Krug, M., Lossner, B., and Ott, T., 1984, Anisomycin blocks the late phase of long-term potentiation in the dentate gyrus of freely moving rats, *Brain Res. Bull.* **13**:39–42.

Lisman, J., 1989, A mechanism for the Hebb and the anti-Hebb processes underlying learning and memory, *Proc. Natl. Acad. Sci. USA* **86**:9574–9578.

Lisman, J. E., and Harris, K. M., 1993, Quantal analysis and synaptic anatomy—Integrating two views of hippocampal plasticity, *Trends Neurosci.* **16**:141–147.

Lovinger, D. M., and Routtenberg, A., 1988, Synapse-specific protein kinase C activation enhances maintenance of long-term potentiation in rat hippocampus, *J. Physiol. (London)* **400**:321–333.

Lynch, G., Larson, J., Kelso, S., Barrioneuvo, G., and Schottler, F., 1983, Intracellular injections of EGTA block induction of hippocampal long-term potentiation, *Nature* **305**:719–721.

Lynch, M. A., Errington, M. L., and Bliss, T. V. P., 1989, Nordihydroguaiaretic acid blocks the synaptic component of long-term potentiation and the associated increases in release of glutamate and arachidonate: An in vivo study in the dentate gyrus of the rat, *Neuroscience* **30**:693–701.

Malenka, R. C., Kauer, J. A., Zucker, R. S., and Nicoll, R. A., 1988, Postsynaptic calcium is sufficient for potentiation of hippocampal synaptic transmission, *Science* **242**:81–84.

Malenka, R. C., Kauer, J. A., Perkel, D. J., Mauk, M. D., Kelly, P. T., Nicoll, R. A., and Waxham, M. N., 1989a, An essential role for postsynaptic calmodulin and protein kinase activity in long-term potentiation, *Nature* **340**:554–557.

Malenka, R. C., Kauer, J. A., Perkel, D. J., and Nicoll, R. A., 1989b, The impact of postsynaptic calcium on synaptic transmission—Its role in long-term potentiation, *Trends Neurosci.* **12**:444–450.

Malinow, R., Schulman, H., and Tsien, R. W., 1989, Inhibition of postsynaptic PKC or CaMKII blocks induction but not expression of LTP, *Science* **245**:862–866.

Miyakawa, H., Ross, W. N., Jaffe, D., Callaway, J. C., Lasser-Ross, N., Lisman, J. E., and Johnston, D., 1992, Synaptically activated increases in Ca^{2+} concentration in hippocampal CA1 pyramidal cells are primarily due to voltage-gated Ca^{2+} channels, *Neuron* **9**:1163–1173.

Mulkey, R. M., and Malenka, R. C., 1992, Mechanisms underlying induction of homosynaptic long-term depression in area CA1 of the hippocampus, *Neuron* **9**:967–975.

Mulkey, R. M., Herron, C. E., and Malenka, R. C., 1993, An essential role for protein phosphatases in hippocampal long-term depression, *Science* **261**:1051–1055.

Mulkey, R. M., Endo, S., Shenolikar, S., and Malenka, R. C., 1994, Involvement of a calcineurin/inhibitor-1 phosphatase cascade in hippocampal long-term depression, *Nature* **369**:486–488.

Muller, D., Joly, M., and Lynch, G., 1988, Contributions of quisqualate and NMDA receptors to the induction and expression of LTP, *Science* **242**:1694–1697.

Musgrave, M. A., Ballyk, B. A., and Goh, J. W., 1993, Coactivation of metabotropic and NMDA receptors is required for LTP induction, *Neuroreport* **4**:171–174.

Nakanishi, S., 1992, Molecular diversity of glutamate receptors and implications for brain function, *Science* **258**:597–603.

Obenaus, A., Mody, I., and Baimbridge, K. G., 1989, Dantrolene-Na (Dantrium) blocks induction of long-term potentiation in hippocampal slices, *Neurosci. Lett.* **98**:172–178.

O'Dell, T. J., Hawkins, R. D., Kandel, E. R., and Arancio, O., 1991a, Tests of the roles of two diffusible substances in long-term potentiation: Evidence for nitric oxide as a possible early retrograde messenger, *Proc. Natl. Acad. Sci. USA* **88**:11285–11289.

O'Dell, T. J., Kandel, E. R., and Grant, S. G. N., 1991b, Long-term potentiation in the hippocampus is blocked by tyrosine kinase inhibitors, *Nature* **353**:558–560.

Otani, S., Marshall, C. J., Tate, W. P., Goddard, G. V., and Abraham, W. C., 1989, Maintenance of long-term potentiation in rat dentate gyrus requires protein synthesis but not messenger RNA synthesis immediately post-tetanization, *Neuroscience* **28**:519–526.

Schuman, E. M., and Madison, D. V., 1991, A requirement for the intracellular messenger nitric oxide in long-term potentiation, *Science* **254**:1503–1506.

Silva, A. J., Stevens, C. F., Tonegawa, S., and Wang, Y., 1992, Deficient hippocampal long-term potentiation in α-calcium-calmodulin kinase II mutant mice, *Science* **257**:201–206.

Stanton, P. K., and Sarvey, J. M., 1984, Blockade of long-term potentiation in rat hippocampal CA1 region by inhibitors of protein synthesis, *J. Neurosci.* **4**:3080–3088.

Tsumoto, T., and Suda, K., 1979, Cross-depression: An electrophysiological manifestation of binocular competition in the developing visual cortex, *Brain Res.* **168**:190–194.

Williams, J. H., Errington, M. L., Lynch, M. A., and Bliss, T. V. P., 1989, Arachidonic acid induces a long-term activity-dependent enhancement of synaptic transmission in the hippocampus, *Nature* **341**:739–742.

Williams, J. H., Li, Y. G., Nayak, A., Errington, M. L., Murphy, K. P. S. J., and Bliss, T. V. P., 1993, The suppression of long-term potentiation in rat hippocampus by inhibitors of nitric oxide synthase is temperature and age dependent, *Neuron* **11**:877–884.

Zalutsky, R. A., and Nicoll, R. A., 1990, Comparison of two forms of long-term potentiation in single hippocampal neurons, *Science* **248**:1619–1624.

12

Mechanisms of Plasticity in the Visual Cortex

Work on LTP suggests a number of transmitters and second messengers that may be involved in plasticity in the hippocampus. Several of these have also been implicated in sensory-dependent plasticity in the visual cortex. We will now review the evidence in the visual cortex for this involvement. We will also review the evidence as to which of the factors might represent a difference between young animals and adults: after all, that is the crucial question in terms of understanding why young animals are plastic and adults are not.

As the reader will see below, the sum of current research suggests that the factors involved in LTP and sensory-dependent plasticity are likely to be similar. Electrical activity leads to glutamate release, which leads to activation of AMPA/kainate, NMDA, and metabotropic glutamate receptors, which leads to activation of second messengers, enzymes, and protein synthesis. Evidence for the visual cortex will be discussed in that order.

I. Electrical Activity

Electrical activity governs sensory-dependent plasticity, as discussed in Chapter 10. The question to be addressed here is: is there anything different about the electrical activity in young animals that affects the maturation of the system?

It is the pattern of electrical activity that is important, rather than the overall level. The pattern of electrical activity distinguishes vertical from horizontal lines, leftward movement from rightward movement, and signals from one eye compared to the other. The pattern of electrical activity is also important before the eyes open. At this stage there are no sensory-dependent signals, but there is an important developmental change that does not occur when electrical activity is abolished by tetrodotoxin, namely the lamination of the lateral geniculate nucleus (Shatz and Stryker, 1988). During this period the ganglion cells in the retina, particularly those near each other, tend to fire with oscillations in synchrony with each other (Wong et al., 1993; Fig. 12.1). The hypothesis is that left eye cells firing in synchrony with each other, and out of

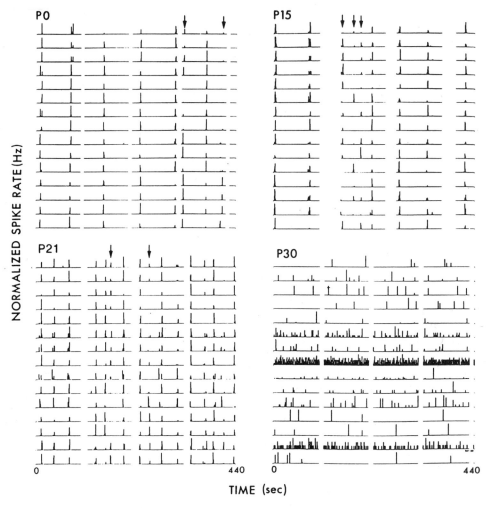

NORMALIZED SPIKE RATE (Hz)

TIME (sec)

FIG. 12.1. Correlated firing between ganglion cells in the ferret at four different ages. Fifteen ganglion cells recorded at each age. Notice correlated firing at P0, P15, and P21, but not at P30. Reprinted with permission from Wong et al. (1993). Copyright Cell Press.

synchrony with right eye cells, lead to the endings of the left and right eye cells in the lateral geniculate nucleus segregating from one another, just as endings from left and right eye projections to layer IV of the cortex segregate from each other later on. The greater tendency for neighboring ganglion cells to fire together may also help to refine the topographic map.

After the eyes open, sensory input becomes important, and the afferents from the lateral geniculate to layer IV of the visual cortex segregate from each other. This process also does not occur when electrical activity is abolished, as pointed out in Chapter 4. Synchrony of activity within each eye would tend to cause the afferents to segregate, and synchrony of activity between the eyes would tend to retain binocularity. Presumably there is substantial synchrony of activity within each eye at 3 weeks of age, to start the process of segregation.

Between 3 and 6 weeks of age, synchrony within each eye is reduced and synchrony between the eyes increases. No quantitative measurement of synchrony of activity within each eye as compared to synchrony between the eyes has been made over this period of time. However, the process seems likely to be organized as suggested above, given the Hebbian mechanism, and the fact that segregation of afferents from the retinas to the lateral geniculate nucleus is complete, while segregation of afferents to the cortex from the lateral geniculate is not.

II. Properties of the Postsynaptic Neuron

The state of depolarization of the postsynaptic neurons within the visual cortex is likely to be important. Both the orientation sensitivity and the ocular dominance of cells can be changed by coupling one stimulus with depolarization of the neuron, and another with hyperpolarization (Fregnac et al., 1992). After several dozen couplings, the cell becomes more responsive to the stimulus coupled with depolarization, and less responsive to the stimulus coupled with hyperpolarization (Fig. 12.2). Indeed, the orientation preference of the cell can be reversed. Moreover, high-frequency stimulation can produce either LTP or LTD in the visual cortex, depending on the state of depolarization of the postsynaptic neuron (Artola et al., 1990; see Fig. 12.3). Putting these two results together suggests that the state of the cellular properties of the neuron may affect what kind of long-term changes result from the visual input impinging on the cortical cell.

A number of cellular properties have been found to change with age in the rat (McCormick and Prince, 1987). The resting potential becomes slightly more hyperpolarized with age. The input resistance drops substantially. Both of these changes could result in the afferent input having a larger effect in young animals. A larger input resistance in young animals will lead to a larger voltage change for the same current input, by Ohm's law. A more depolarized resting potential will bring the membrane potential closer to threshold for action potentials, and also closer to the potential required to activate NMDA currents, so that a smaller change in voltage will activate these. Moreover, the inhibitory transmitter GABA actually excites neurons in young animals, leading to a calcium influx, because its reversal potential is more positive than the membrane potential of the cell at that age (Yuste and Katz, 1991; Lin et al., 1994). Unfortunately, these experiments have not been carried out in the cat visual cortex, where the time course of the critical period is well defined. Consequently, we do not know if these changes are complete before the critical period, or take place during and after it.

III. NMDA Receptors

Kleinschmidt et al. (1987) were the first to show that an NMDA antagonist will reduce sensory-dependent plasticity. They infused APV directly into the visual cortex with an Alzet osmotic minipump, then closed the eyelid of one

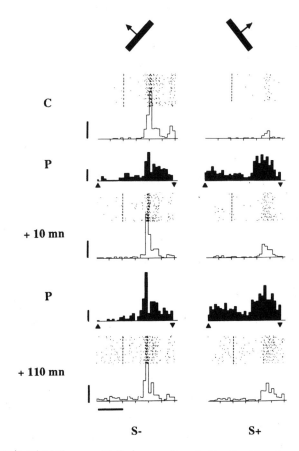

FIG. 12.2. Change in orientation sensitivity by coupling of stimuli with polarization of the cell. In the control situation (C), the cell preferred movement up and to the left. After pairing movement up right with depolarization, and movement up left with hyperpolarization, this orientation preference was reversed (P). Ten minutes later, the cell had reverted to its original orientation preference (10 mn). Two hours after a second pairing (110 mn), some shift in orientation preference persisted. Reprinted with permission from Fregnac *et al.* (1992).

eye to test the effects of monocular deprivation. The ocular dominance shift that normally occurs after monocular deprivation was smaller than usual (Fig. 12.4). Also, the receptive fields of the cells were not as specific for the orientation and direction of movement of the stimulus as usual. Thus, several processes that normally occur during development were disrupted.

In interpreting this result, it is important to know whether APV reduces the activity in the visual cortex so much that the treatment is essentially like infusing TTX. Barbara Gordon and I repeated the experiment with a different technique—intramuscular infusion of an NMDA channel blocker that can cross the blood–brain barrier (MK-801)—and concluded that ocular dominance shifts are reduced by about the same amount as in the Kleinschmidt *et al.* experiment without abolishing activity in the visual cortex. Activity was reduced (it was at least 50–75% of normal for at least three-fourths of the time)

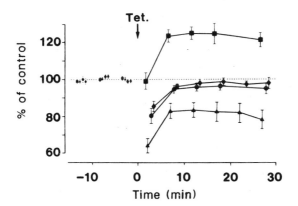

FIG. 12.3. LTP and LTD in slices of rat visual cortex. A tetanus (a burst of high-frequency stimulation) was applied at time 0. In normal conditions, there was no long-term effect. With a low level of the GABA antagonist bicuculline (0.1–0.2 μM), which blocks inhibitory signals and depolarizes the neuron, the tetanus produced LTD (▲) and with a higher level of bicuculline (0.3 μM) the tetanus produced LTP (■). Reprinted with permission from Artola, A., Brocher, S., and Singer, W., 1990. Different voltage-dependent thresholds for inducing long-term depression and long-term potentiation in slices of rat visual cortex, *Nature* **347**:69–72. Copyright 1990, MacMillan Magazines Limited.

FIG. 12.4. Ocular dominance histograms from kittens infused with APV into the experimental hemisphere (A, C, and E) compared to histograms from the control hemisphere (B, D, and F). A and B dark-reared until treatment, C–F reared normally. A and C treated with 50 mM APV, E with 5 mM. The differences between A and B, and between C and D were substantially greater than the difference seen in monocularly deprived animals not treated with an antagonist, between the hemispheres ipsilateral and contralateral to the open eye. Fewer cells were specific for the orientation of the stimulus in APV-treated animals. Thus, treatment with APV reduced both the ocular dominance shift and the orientation specificity. Reprinted with permission from Kleinschmidt *et al., Science* **238**:355–358. Copyright 1987, American Association for the Advancement of Science.

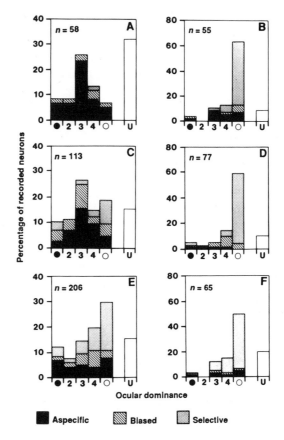

but it was not abolished as it is by TTX (see Daw, 1994). However, one should point out that the ocular dominance shift was also reduced, and not totally abolished in either of these experiments. The conclusion is that NMDA receptors play some role in plasticity in the visual cortex, but the nature of that role needs to be elucidated.

As pointed out in Chapter 10, the total number of NMDA receptors in the visual cortex varies with age, and the number peaks at the same time that the critical period for shifts in ocular dominance peaks (Gordon *et al.*, 1991). There are still substantial numbers of NMDA receptors in the adult visual cortex. These are found primarily in layers II and III. Presumably they are there for some other function—either the normal processing of visual information, or some form of plasticity other than ocular dominance shifts.

One can also measure a physiological parameter that represents the contribution of NMDA receptors to the visual response. One does this by recording from cells in the visual cortex and iontophoresing the NMDA antagonist APV. The amount by which the visual response is reduced represents the NMDA contribution to the visual response, in relation to the contribution from AMPA/kainate receptors. This NMDA contribution remains high in layers II and III of the visual cortex at all ages (Fox *et al.*, 1989). However, it drops in layers IV, V, and VI between 3 and 6 weeks of age (Fig. 12.5). This is the period when ocular dominance columns are segregating in layer IV.

Rearing in the dark is known to postpone the critical period for ocular dominance changes in the visual cortex (see Chapter 10). Rearing in the dark also postpones the reduction in the NMDA contribution to the visual response in layers IV, V, and VI (Fox *et al.*, 1992): even after several months in the dark, the contribution remains high (Fig. 12.6). If animals are brought into the light after being in the dark until 6 weeks of age, then the reduction in the NMDA

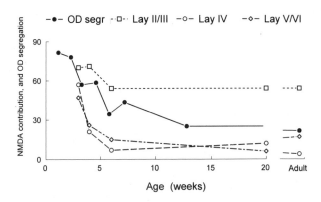

FIG. 12.5. Change in NMDA contribution to the visual response with age, compared with ocular dominance segregation. NMDA contribution to the visual response was calculated by recording the response from a single cell, iontophoresing the NMDA antagonist APV, and observing the reduction in response: values were taken from a number of single cells and averaged to give the points in the graph. Ocular dominance segregation index was calculated from grain counts from [³H]proline transported from one eye to layer IV in the visual cortex (LeVay *et al.*, 1978). Counts were scaled to use the same scale as NMDA contribution to the visual response (100 represents complete overlap, and 0 represents complete segregation). Reprinted with permission from *Investigative Ophthalmology and Visual Science*, Daw (1994).

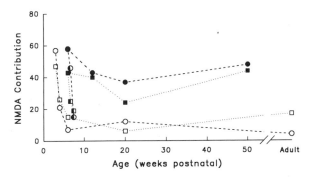

FIG. 12.6. Effect of rearing in the dark on the NMDA contribution to the visual response. NMDA contribution remains high in dark-reared animals in layer IV (●) and layers V and VI (■), compared with animals reared in the light (○ and □). When animals are reared in the dark until 6 weeks of age, then brought into the light, the drop in the NMDA contribution to the visual response proceeds (◑ and ◪). Reprinted with permission from the *Journal of Neurophysiology*, Czepita and Daw (1994).

contribution to the visual response proceeds. Thus, the change in the NMDA contribution to the visual response is definitely under the control of light.

This drop in the NMDA contribution to the visual response reflects, among other things, a change in the properties of the NMDA receptors (Carmignoto and Vicini, 1992). EPSPs produced by NMDA receptors in the rat visual cortex become shorter as the animal gets older. This occurs because the NMDA channels are open for a shorter period of time in the older animals. This change in the kinetics of the NMDA receptor can also be delayed by rearing in the dark.

NMDA receptors have also been shown to have an effect on the morphology of neurons in the visual system. Ocular dominance stripes can be created in the frog tectum by implanting a third eye. Application of NMDA sharpens these stripes, while application of the NMDA antagonist APV blurs them (Cline *et al.*, 1987); in other words, activation of NMDA receptors affects the pattern of terminals of the retinal afferents to the tectum. Moreover, application of NMDA to the ferret lateral geniculate can affect the formation of dendritic spines over a period of hours (Rocha and Sur, 1994).

Thus, NMDA receptors fulfill several of the criteria for a factor or substance that is crucial for plasticity in the visual cortex. They are activated by the sensory signals that govern plasticity. Antagonists to NMDA receptors reduce plasticity. There are more of them in the visual cortex at the peak of the critical period for plasticity than later in development. Their contribution to the visual response declines as ocular dominance changes occur. In summary, because they are more active during the critical period, NMDA receptors may allow young animals to be plastic, while adults are not.

IV. Metabotropic Glutamate Receptors

There are at least seven types of metabotropic glutamate receptor. Some affect inositol phosphates, some affect cyclic AMP, and one affects both. The production of inositol phosphates by the metabotropic agonist ibotenate peaks with the critical period (Dudek and Bear, 1989). There are increases in cAMP driven by metabotropic glutamate agonists that vary with age in visual cortex, but not decreases (Flavin *et al.*, 1994). These two pieces of evidence suggest that the metabotropic glutamate receptors of interest are the ones that affect inositol phosphates, namely mGluR1 and mGluR5, and the one that produces increases in cAMP, which may also be mGluR1.

Immunocytochemistry shows that expression of these metabotropic glutamate receptors changes with age (Reid *et al.*, 1995). The amount of mGluR1 declines with age after the peak of the critical period. The laminar pattern of mGluR5 changes: early in life, it is widespread from layers III to VI, and during the critical period it becomes confined to layer IV (Fig. 12.7). This distribution corresponds to the endings of afferents projecting from the lateral geniculate nucleus, which are also widespread early on, and then become confined to layer IV.

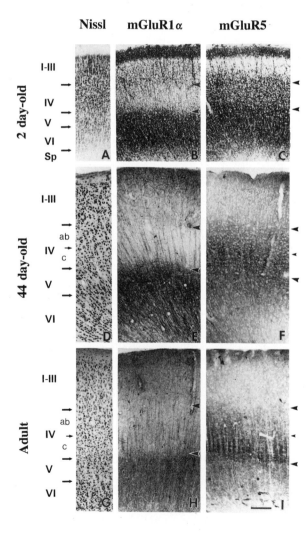

FIG. 12.7. Changes in staining with antibodies for mGluR1 and mGluR5 with age. The laminar pattern for mGluR1 does not change, but the staining is reduced after the peak of the critical period. The laminar pattern for mGluR5 does change: early, it is widespread, and during the critical period it becomes confined to layer IV. Reprinted with permission from Reid, S. N. M., Romano, C., Hughes, T., and Daw, N. W., 1995, Immunohistochemical study of two phosphoinositide-linked metabotropic glutamate receptors (mGluR1α and mGluR5) in the cat visual cortex before, during and after the peak of the critical period for eye-specific connections, *J. Comp. Neurol.* **355:** 470–478. Copyright 1995, John Wiley & Sons, Inc.

We do not know if a metabotropic antagonist will reduce or abolish plasticity. Antagonists available before 1990 were not very specific. The antagonist used (2-amino-3-phosphonopropionate) did reduce plasticity when infused directly into the visual cortex, but the results were variable (Bear and Dudek, 1991). The more specific antagonist that is now available (RS-α-methyl-4-carboxyphenylglycine) is unfortunately not very potent. It does not block ocular dominance changes when infused into the cortex (Hensch and Stryker, 1994); however, it may not be a good antagonist for the effect of metabotropic glutamate receptors on increases in cAMP (Flavin et al., 1994). Thus, the evidence for involvement of metabotropic glutamate receptors in ocular dominance plasticity is not as clear as the evidence for NMDA receptors. Metabotropic glutamate receptors change during development with a time course that is related to the critical period, but whether they are a crucial factor in the pathway has not been established.

V. Calcium

Calcium is likely to be involved in plasticity, if NMDA receptors are, because NMDA receptors allow calcium to enter the cell (Takahashi et al., 1993). The amount of calcium that is taken up by cells in the visual cortex in response to NMDA decreases with age (Feldman et al., 1990). This decrease can be accounted for largely by the decrease in NMDA receptors that also occurs over the same time period. The effect of dark-rearing on this calcium uptake is complicated. In animals reared in the dark to 6 weeks of age, the basal level of calcium uptake is increased (i.e., non-NMDA-dependent calcium uptake), whereas the uptake related to NMDA receptors is decreased, compared with normal animals of the same age. At this age, light-reared animals are more plastic than dark-reared (Mower, 1991), and therefore calcium entry related to NMDA receptors is consistent with the idea that NMDA receptors are important in regulating plasticity. Animals were not reared to 12–20 weeks of age, which produces dark-reared animals that are more plastic than light-reared, and might therefore show a larger calcium uptake in the dark-reared than in the normal animals. Thus, it is not yet clear if there is any change in calcium entry from NMDA receptors, as opposed to the number of NMDA receptors, that can be related to plasticity.

Binding sites for the voltage-sensitive calcium channels that are marked by 1,4-dihydropyridine decrease in number between 14 and 28 days of age, and change their distribution from lower layer IV to the upper cortical layers (Bode-Greuel and Singer, 1988). Since there is no sensory-dependent plasticity at 14 days of age, and substantial plasticity at 28 days of age, this change must reflect some developmental process other than sensory-dependent plasticity.

No one has attempted to find out if blocking of those calcium changes in the postsynaptic cell that are related to glutamate receptor activity will also block visual plasticity. This is because the experiment would be impossible to interpret. To affect ocular dominance changes, calcium changes would have to be blocked in a large number of cells over a long period of time, and this would have an effect on a number of other processes in the cell, such as the firing of action potentials. Thus, the treatment would be likely to inactivate the cortex altogether, like TTX. However, injection of calcium chelators into the post-synaptic cell does block induction of long-term potentiation (Kimura et al., 1990) and probably also long-term depression (Brocher et al., 1992; Kato, 1993) in the visual cortex, as it does in the hippocampus.

In summary, changes in calcium levels are almost certainly involved in plasticity in the visual cortex, because NMDA receptors are involved, and NMDA receptors let calcium into the cell. There are changes in the control of calcium levels in the cell with age. Some are related to changes in the NMDA system, which will let less calcium into the cell as the number of NMDA receptors declines with age. The non-NMDA-dependent changes in calcium levels that have so far been studied have the wrong time course to be correlated with plasticity, peaking before the critical period for sensory-dependent plasticity starts. Thus, there is no evidence at the present time that the calcium system itself, as opposed to factors that control it, is most active when plasticity is highest.

VI. Other Second Messengers, Enzymes, and Proteins

The enzyme that has been most studied in the visual cortex is protein kinase C (PKC). PKC is activated through phosphoinositol hydrolysis by several neurotransmitter receptors, including metabotropic glutamate receptors.

Activity of PKC in both cytosol and membranes changes with age (Sheu et al., 1990). The change in cytosol PKC activity is particularly pronounced, and follows the critical period for plasticity quite closely (Fig. 12.8). There is a large rise between 1 and 3 weeks of age, when the critical period starts, a peak at 7 weeks of age, just after the peak of the critical period, and a substantial decline between then and 1 year of age, when the critical period is largely over. This general time course is confirmed with an antibody against PKC isozymes II and III (Stichel and Singer, 1989). The time course seen with polyclonal antibodies directed against PKC is different, with a general decrease in staining between 10 and 90 days of age, but these antibodies do show that the staining decrease occurs in layer IV before it occurs in other layers (Jia et al., 1990). Taking into account the biochemical results for the overall activity, and the immunohisto-chemistry for the layering pattern, the conclusion is that PKC follows the critical period for plasticity quite closely, both in terms of overall activity and in terms of the property of ocular dominance plasticity that it decreases in layer IV before it decreases in other layers.

A number of other enzymes and proteins have been investigated, but none has yet been shown to have activity and location changes that parallel the critical period closely, as PKC does. Calcium/calmodulin-dependent protein kinase II (CaM-KII) shows laminar changes during development, but there is substantial immunoreactivity in the adult (Jia et al., 1992). This is to be expected of a protein that is a major component of postsynaptic densities, and therefore plays a role in synaptic function at all ages. However, mice that do not express the gene for CaM-KII show ocular dominance changes (Gordon et al., 1994), implying that CaM-KII is not a crucial factor in ocular dominance plas-

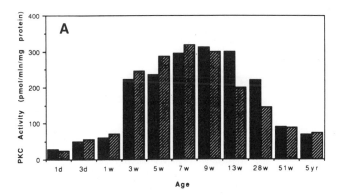

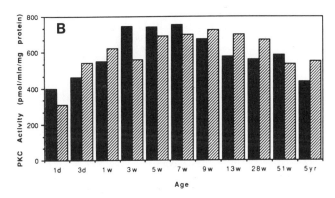

FIG. 12.8. Changes in PKC activity with age in cat visual cortex. (A) Cytosol PKC activity. (B) Membrane PKC activity. Two subjects measured at each age. Reprinted with kind permission from Sheu, F. S., Kasamatsu, T., and Routtenberg, A., 1990, Protein kinase C activity and substrate (F1/GAP-43) phosphorylation in developing cat visual cortex, *Brain Res.* **524:**144–148. Copyright 1990, Elsevier Science, Ltd., The Boulevard, Langford Lane, Kidlington OX5 1GB, UK.

ticity. The enzyme 5'-nucleotidase is concentrated in layer IV, with a patchy appearance between 4 and 6 weeks of age, and is found in all layers in the adult (Schoen *et al.*, 1990). This enzyme faces the cell exterior, and converts nucleotides to the membrane-permeable adenosine. The expression of this enzyme could be related to the segregation of left and right eye input between 4 and 6 weeks of age, but how it might act is a matter of speculation. The glial protein S100β is found in layer IV between weeks 2 and 5, then increases disproportionately in other layers, so that layer IV is stained less than other layers in the adult (Dyck *et al.*, 1993). More experiments will be needed to interpret this finding. Calcineurin is a calcium-dependent, calmodulin-stimulated protein phosphatase which has a particularly high concentration in the brain. LTP in the visual cortex is enhanced by a calcineurin inhibitor (Funauchi *et al.*, 1994). Immunocytochemistry for calcineurin shows a high expression in cell bodies in layer IV at the peak of the critical period, and high expression in cell bodies in layers II and III in the adult (Goto *et al.*, 1993). This pattern is similar to the distribution of NMDA receptors; calcineurin could likewise play a role in ocular dominance plasticity, with an additional role in the adult. Thus, evidence for the involvement of these proteins is intriguing, but incomplete. In each case, many more experiments are required.

Two exciting new techniques that can be used to identify proteins that could be involved in plasticity are subtractive hybridization and immunosuppression (Prasad and Cynader, 1994; Kind et al., 1994). These techniques have been used to identify mRNA and antigens that are in high abundance in 30-day-old kittens compared to adults. Two percent of molecules are in this category, and include proteins involved in cell–cell interaction, cellular remodeling, neurofilament assembly, neurotransmitter release, energy metabolism, RNA processing, and protein synthesis. Which of the proteins are specifically related to plasticity will require considerable further experiments.

VII. Modulatory Neurotransmitters

The factors considered so far are those that may be directly along the series of reactions between the electrical activity that carries the visual signals to the cortex, and the protein changes that produce alterations in axons, dendrites, and synapses. Steps along this series of reactions can also be affected, or "gated," by signals coming in from other sources. These gating signals can affect the state of depolarization of neurons in the visual cortex, or act on the same second messengers (e.g., inositol phosphates, calcium, cyclic AMP) and enzymes that are affected by signals directly along the pathway.

The four main modulatory pathways to the visual cortex use acetylcholine, noradrenaline, serotonin, and dopamine. Acetylcholine signals come from the basal forebrain, noradrenaline signals from the locus coeruleus, serotonin signals from the raphe nuclei, and dopamine signals from the brain stem. Activity in these pathways carries signals about the general state of the animal, such as state of attention, and the sleep/wake cycle.

At one point it was thought that abolition of noradrenaline input to the visual cortex would affect ocular dominance plasticity (Kasamatsu and Pettigrew, 1979). This turned out to be related to nonspecific effects of the drug used (see Daw et al., 1985; Gordon et al., 1988). However, lesions of the noradrenaline and acetylcholine systems together can affect ocular dominance plasticity (Bear and Singer, 1986; Gordon et al., 1990) and so can antagonists that affect the acetylcholine system alone (Gu and Singer, 1993). The result, as with the NMDA antagonist APV, is a reduction in ocular dominance shifts rather than an abolition of ocular dominance shifts.

The interpretation of these results is complicated. There are several receptors for both noradrenaline and acetylcholine. Stimulation of the locus coeruleus activates both α- and β-adrenergic receptors in the visual cortex. The influence of α-adrenergic receptors is excitatory, while the influence of β-adrenergic receptors is inhibitory (Sato et al., 1989). Most of the acetylcholine receptors are muscarinic, but there is a multiplicity of muscarinic receptors with different mechanisms of action. For example, M_1 receptors mediate phosphoinositide metabolism, whereas M_2 receptors inhibit adenylate cyclase (see Prusky and Cynader, 1990). A comprehensive view of how these two modulatory transmitters interact with the signals mediated by glutamate remains to be worked out.

When one looks at the laminar pattern of transmitter receptors, and how it changes with age, there is an intriguing pattern (Fig. 12.9). AMPA, kainate, and GABA receptors do not change much with age. AMPA receptors are highest in superficial and deep layers, kainate receptors highest in deep layers, and GABA receptors highest in layer IV at all ages (Cynader *et al.*, 1991). On the other hand, many of the modulatory transmitters are high in layer IV at an early age, then move to superficial layers later on. This is true of acetylcholine muscarinic receptors (Fig. 12.10), and adrenergic α1 and β receptors. Moreover, this rearrangement is prevented by removal of the afferent visual input (Liu *et al.*, 1994). Thus, the location of these transmitter receptors depends on the sensory input.

Some serotonin receptors have a staining pattern that follows columns in the cortex as well as layers. Serotonin 1C receptors are expressed transiently between 4 and 12 weeks of age in layer IV in a patchy distribution (Dyck and Cynader, 1993; Fig. 12.11). Serotonin 2 receptors are also found in patches in layer IV, peaking at a later age. The patches are complementary to cytochrome oxidase staining (Dyck and Cynader, 1993). Since cytochrome oxidase staining is centered on ocular dominance columns, the serotonin 1C receptors are at the boundaries of those columns. Zinc colocalizes with serotonin 1C, and acetylcholinesterase with cytochrome oxidase. Thus, serotonin 1C receptors may be related to the formation of ocular dominance columns.

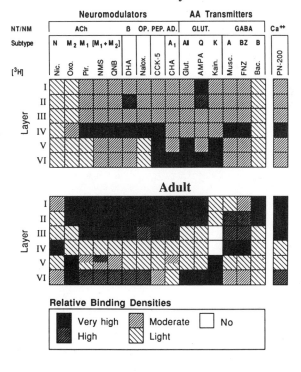

FIG. 12.9. Rearrangement of neurotransmitter receptors in cat visual cortex between young animals and adults. The top row of the figure lists the neurotransmitters: acetylcholine (ACh), beta-adrenergic (β), opiates (OP), peptides (PEP), adenosine (AD), glutamate (GLUT), and GABA. Receptor subtypes are listed in the next row, and ligands in the subsequent row. There is a substantial redistribution from layer IV to superficial layers for neuromodulators. Reprinted with permission from Cynader, Shaw, van Huizen, and Prusky, in: *Development of the Visual System*, MIT Press, © 1991 Massachusetts Institute of Technology.

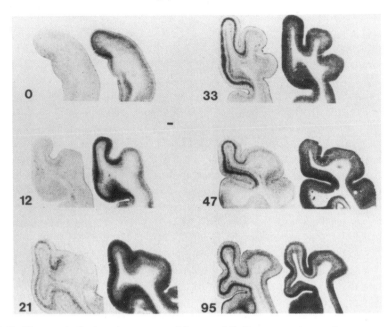

FIG. 12.10. Changes in the layering pattern of the acetylcholine muscarinic and nicotinic receptors as a function of age in cat visual cortex. Ages shown at bottom left of each pair of photographs. In each pair, binding of [³H]nicotine is on the left, and binding of [³H]QNB for muscarinic receptors is on the right. Nicotinic receptors appear at day 21, and are always found in layer IV. Muscarinic receptors are found in layer IV at day 0, move to superficial layers by day 21, and are found in superficial and deep layers in the adult. Reprinted with permission from Cynader, Shaw, van Huizen, and Prusky, in: *Development of the Visual System*, MIT Press, © 1991 Massachusetts Institute of Technology.

These experiments show that cause and effect in the interactions between the sensory input, carried by glutamate, and the modulatory or "gating" signals, carried by acetylcholine, noradrenaline, serotonin, and dopamine, is complicated. Abolition of sensory input can affect the distribution of receptors for the modulatory neurotransmitters in the cortex. At the same time, it seems likely that abolition of some of the modulatory input can affect ocular dominance, which is determined by the arrangement of sensory endings. The purpose of such a two-way flow of effects is intriguing and unexplained.

VIII. Growth Factors

A number of different receptors for various growth factors have been found in the visual system (Allendorfer *et al.*, 1994), but so far not very many functional experiments have been carried out. Two groups have observed the effect of infusion of nerve growth factor (NGF) on monocular deprivation. One found that NGF prevents the shift in ocular dominance that normally occurs during the critical period (Carmignoto *et al.*, 1993). Their hypothesis was that NGF causes sprouting of nerve terminals, consequently endings from the deprived eye did not retract. The other group found that NGF promotes a shift in ocular

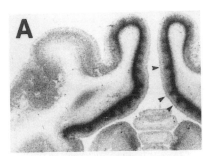

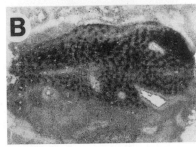

FIG. 12.11. Pattern of serotonin 2C binding in 50-day-old cat visual cortex. (A) Vertical section showing continuous labeling in layer V, and patchy labeling in layer IV. (B) Horizontal section showing the patches where the section goes through layer IV. Reprinted with permission from Dyck and Cynader (1993).

dominance toward the deprived eye after monocular deprivation in the adult (Gu *et al.*, 1994). These somewhat contradictory findings have not been explained. NGF is known to promote the growth of acetylcholine cells projecting from the basal forebrain to the cortex. Quite possibly, NGF affects acetylcholine modulation of visual signals, and other growth factors, such as brain-derived nerve growth factor (BDNF), act more directly on the geniculocortical pathway (Cabelli *et al.*, 1994).

IX. Hormones

Cortisol reduces ocular dominance shifts after monocular deprivation (Daw *et al.*, 1991). The hypothesis behind this experiment was that the rise in cortisol that occurs just before puberty, known as adrenarche, might play a role in ending the critical period. However, the experiment was done in cats, and it was found that cats do not have a rise in plasma concentrations of cortisol before puberty, as humans do. There could be a change in cortisol receptors, but this has not been tested. Interpretation of this experiment is thus uncertain.

X. Feedback Factors

There is very little evidence on feedback factors in visual plasticity. The effect of nitric oxide synthase inhibitors on ocular dominance plasticity has been tested by two groups (Gillespie *et al.*, 1993; Daw *et al.*, 1994). In neither case did the inhibitors reduce plasticity substantially.

XI. Summary

This chapter shows that, when one considers the criteria listed in Chapter 10 for a factor that is crucially involved in plasticity in the visual cortex, very few factors have been adequately tested. To some extent, NMDA receptors fulfill all three criteria. Their concentration peaks with the critical period; their contribution to the visual response declines with ocular dominance segregation; dark-rearing postpones this change; and application of NMDA antagonists reduces ocular dominance plasticity.

Metabotropic glutamate receptors produce increases in phosphoinositides and cAMP that follow the critical period, but it is not clear whether metabotropic glutamate antagonists affect ocular dominance plasticity. Calcium that enters the cell as a result of NMDA receptors changes with age, but this is probably related simply to the change in the number of NMDA receptors. Calcium that enters the cell from voltage-dependent calcium channels is reduced before the critical period for sensory-dependent plasticity starts. As far as proteins and enzymes are concerned, few quantitative measurements have been made. Only PKC has been shown to follow the critical period closely, in terms of both overall concentration and layering pattern, in experiments that have been completed to date. Much work remains to be done.

References

Allendorfer, K. L., Cabelli, R. J., Escandon, E., Kaplan, D. R., Nikolics, K., and Shatz, C. J., 1994, Regulation of neurotrophin receptors during the maturation of the mammalian visual system, *J. Neurosci.* **14**:1795–1811.

Artola, A., Brocher, S., and Singer, W., 1990, Different voltage-dependent thresholds for inducing long-term depression and long-term potentiation in slices of rat visual cortex, *Nature* **347**: 69–72.

Bear, M. F., and Dudek, S. M., 1991, Stimulation of phosphoinositide turnover by excitatory amino acids: Pharmacology, development, and role in visual cortical plasticity, *Ann. N.Y. Acad. Sci.* **627**:42–56.

Bear, M. F., and Singer, W., 1986, Modulation of visual cortical plasticity by acetylcholine and noradrenaline, *Nature* **320**:172–176.

Bode-Greuel, K. M., and Singer, W., 1988, Developmental changes of the distribution of binding sites for organic Ca^{++} channel blockers in cat visual cortex, *Brain Res.* **70**:266–275.

Brocher, S., Artola, A., and Singer, W., 1992, Intracellular injection of Ca^{2+} chelators blocks induction of long-term depression in rat visual cortex, *Proc. Natl. Acad. Sci. USA* **89**:123–127.

Cabelli, R. J., Radeke, M. J., Wright, A., Allendorfer, K. L., Feinstein, S. C., and Shatz, C. J., 1994, Developmental patterns of localization of full-length and truncated TRKB proteins in the mammalian visual system, *Soc. Neurosci. Abstr.* **20**:37.

Carmignoto, G., and Vicini, S., 1992, Activity-dependent decrease in NMDA receptor responses during development of the visual cortex, *Science* **258**:1007–1011.

Carmignoto, G., Canella, R., Candeo, P., Comelli, M. C., and Maffei, L., 1993, Effects of nerve growth factor on neuronal plasticity of the kitten visual cortex, *J. Physiol. (London)* **464**:343–360.

Cline, H. T., Debski, E. A., and Constantine-Paton, M., 1987, N-methyl-D-aspartate antagonist desegregates eye-specific stripes, *Proc. Natl. Acad. Sci. USA* **84**:4342–4345.

Cynader, M. S., Shaw, C., van Huizen, F., and Prusky, G. T., 1991, Redistribution of neurotransmitter receptors and the mechanism of cortical developmental plasticity, in: *Development of the Visual System* (D. M. Lam and C. J. Shatz, eds.), MIT Press, Cambridge, MA, pp. 253–265.

Daw, N. W., 1994, Mechanisms of plasticity in the visual cortex, *Invest. Ophthalmol. Vis. Sci.* **35**:4168–4179.

Daw, N. W., Videen, T. O., Parkinson, D., and Rader, R. K., 1985, DSP-4 (N-(2-chloroethyl)-N-ethyl-2-bromobenzylamine) depletes noradrenaline in kitten visual cortex without altering the effects of visual deprivation, *J. Neurosci.* **5:**1925–1933.

Daw, N. W., Sato, H., Fox, K., Carmichael, T., and Gingerich, R., 1991, Cortisol reduces plasticity in the kitten visual cortex, *J. Neurobiol.* **22:**158–168.

Daw, N. W., Reid, S. N. M., and Czepita, D., 1994, Infusion of a nitric oxide synthase inhibitor in vivo reduces the ocular dominance shift after monocular deprivation, *Invest. Ophthalmol. Vis. Sci.* **35(Suppl.):**1773.

Dudek, S. M., and Bear, M. F., 1989, A biochemical correlate of the critical period for synaptic modification in the visual cortex, *Science* **246:**673–675.

Dyck, R. H., and Cynader, M. S., 1993, Autoradiographic localization of serotonin receptor subtypes in cat visual cortex: Transient regional, laminar and columnar distributions during postnatal development, *J. Neurosci.* **13:**4316–4338.

Dyck, R. H., and Cynader, M. S., 1993, An interdigitated columnar mosaic of cytochrome oxidase, zinc and neurotransmitter-related molecules in cat and monkey visual cortex, *Proc. Natl. Acad. Sci. USA* **90:**9066–9099.

Dyck, R. H., Van Eldik, L. J., and Cynader, M. S., 1993, Immunohistochemical localization of the S-100β protein in postnatal cat visual cortex: Spatial and temporal patterns of expression in cortical and subcortical glia, *Dev. Brain Res.* **72:**181–192.

Feldman, D., Sherin, J. E., Press, W. A., and Bear, M. F., 1990, N-methyl-D-aspartate-evoked calcium uptake by kitten visual cortex maintained in vitro, *Exp. Brain Res.* **80:**252–259.

Flavin, H. J., Daw, N. W., Gregory, D., and Reid, S. N. M., 1994, Metabotropic glutamate receptor stimulated cAMP is implicated in visual cortical plasticity, *Soc. Neurosci. Abstr.* **20:**1171.

Fox, K., Sato, H., and Daw, N. W., 1989, The location and function of NMDA receptors in cat and kitten visual cortex, *J. Neurosci.* **9:**2443–2454.

Fox, K., Daw, N. W., Sato, H., and Czepita, D., 1992, The effect of visual experience on development of NMDA receptor synaptic transmission in kitten visual cortex, *J. Neurosci.* **12:**2672–2684.

Fregnac, Y., Schulz, D., Thorpe, S., and Bienenstock, E., 1992, Cellular analogs of visual cortical epigenesis. I. Plasticity of orientation selectivity, *J. Neurosci.* **12:**1280–1300, 1301–1318.

Funauchi, M., Haruta, H., and Tsumoto, T., 1994, Effects of an inhibitor for calcium/calmodulin-dependent protein phosphatase, calcineurin, on induction of long-term potentiation in rat visual cortex, *Neurosci. Res.* **19:**269–278.

Gillespie, D. C., Ruthazer, S., Dawson, T. M., Snyder, S. H., and Stryker, M. P., 1993, Nitric oxide synthase inhibition does not prevent ocular dominance plasticity in cat visual cortex, *Soc. Neurosci. Abstr.* **19:**893.

Gordon, B., Allen, E. E., and Trombley, P. Q., 1988, The role of norepinephrine in plasticity of visual cortex, *Prog. Neurobiol.* **30:**171–191.

Gordon, B., Mitchell, B., Mohtadi, K., Roth, E., Tseng, Y., and Turk, F., 1990, Lesions of nonvisual inputs affect plasticity, norepinephrine content and acetylcholine content of visual cortex, *J. Neurophysiol.* **64:**1851–1860.

Gordon, B., Daw, N. W., and Parkinson, D., 1991, The effect of age on binding of MK-801 in the cat visual cortex, *Dev. Brain Res.* **62:**61–67.

Gordon, J. A., Silva, A., Morris, R., Stewart, C., Silver, I., Tokugawa, Y., and Stryker, M. P., 1994, Plasticity in mouse visual cortex: Critical period and effects of αCaMKII and Thy-I mutations, *Soc. Neurosci. Abstr.* **20:**405.

Goto, S., Singer, W., and Gu, Q., 1993, Immunocytochemical localization of calcineurin in the adult and developing primary visual cortex of cats, *Exp. Brain Res.* **96:**377–386.

Gu, Q., and Singer, W., 1993, Effects of intracortical infusion of anticholinergic drugs on neuronal plasticity in kitten striate cortex, *Eur. J. Neurosci.* **5:**475–485.

Gu, Q., Liu, Y., and Cynader, M. S., 1994, Nerve growth factor-induced ocular dominance plasticity in adult cat visual cortex, *Proc. Natl. Acad. Sci. USA* **91:**8408–8412.

Hensch, T. K., and Stryker, M. P., 1994, Postsynaptic metabotropic glutamate receptors do not mediate ocular dominance plasticity, *Soc. Neurosci. Abstr.* **20:**216.

Jia, W. G., Beaulieu, C., Huang, F. L., and Cynader, M. S., 1990, Protein kinase C immunoreactivity in kitten visual cortex is developmentally regulated and input-dependent, *Dev. Brain Res.* **57:**209–222.

Jia, W. G., Beaulieu, C., Liu, Y. L., and Cynader, M. S., 1992, Calcium calmodulin dependent kinase II in cat visual cortex and its development, *Dev. Neurosci.* **14:**238–246.

Kasamatsu, T., and Pettigrew, J. D., 1979, Preservation of binocularity after monocular deprivation in the striate cortex of kittens treated with 6-hydroxydopamine, *J. Comp. Neurol.* **185:**139–162.

Kato, N., 1993, Dependence of long-term depression on postsynaptic metabotropic glutamate receptors in visual cortex, *Proc. Natl. Acad. Sci. USA* **90:**3650–3654.

Kimura, F., Tsumoto, T., Nishigori, A., and Yoshimura, Y., 1990, Long-term depression but not potentiation is induced in Ca^{2+}-chelated visual cortex neurons, *Neuroreport* **1:**65–68.

Kind, P., Blakemore, C., Fryer, H., and Hockfield, S., 1994, Identification of proteins downregulated during the postnatal development of the cat visual cortex, *Cereb. Cortex* **4:**361–375.

Kleinschmidt, A., Bear, M. F., and Singer, W., 1987, Blockade of "NMDA" receptors disrupts experience-dependent plasticity of kitten striate cortex, *Science* **238:**355–358.

LeVay, S., Stryker, M. P., and Shatz, C. J., 1978, Ocular dominance columns and their development in layer IV of the cat's visual cortex: A quantitative study, *J. Comp. Neurol.* **179:**223–244.

Lin, M. H., Takahashi, M. P., Takahashi, Y., and Tsumoto, T., 1994, Intracellular calcium increase induced by GABA in visual cortex of fetal and neonatal rats and its disappearance with development, *Neurosci. Res.* **20:**85–94.

Liu, Y., Jia, W., Gu, Q., and Cynader, M. S., 1994, Involvement of muscarinic acetylcholine receptors in regulation of kitten visual cortex plasticity, *Dev. Brain Res.* **79:**63–71.

McCormick, D. A., and Prince, D. A., 1987, Post-natal development of electrophysiological properties of rat cerebral cortical pyramidal neurons, *J. Physiol. (London)* **383:**743–762.

Mower, G. D., 1991, The effect of dark rearing on the time course of the critical period in cat visual cortex, *Dev. Brain Res.* **58:**151–158.

Prasad, S. S., and Cynader, M. S., 1994, Identification of cDNA clones expressed selectively during the critical period for visual cortex development by subtractive hybridization, *Brain Res.* **639:**73–84.

Prusky, G. T., and Cynader, M. S., 1990, The distribution of M1 and M2 muscarinic acetylcholine receptor subtypes in the developing cat visual cortex, *Dev. Brain Res.* **56:**1–12.

Reid, S. N. M., Romano, C., Hughes, T., and Daw, N. W., 1995, Immunohistochemical study of two phosphoinositide-linked metabotropic glutamate receptors (mGluR1α and mGluR5) in the cat visual cortex before, during and after the peak of the critical period for eye-specific connections, *J. Comp. Neurol.* **355:**1–8.

Rocha, M., and Sur, M., 1994, Rapid acquisition of dendritic spines by visual thalamic neurons after blockade of NMDA receptors, *Soc. Neurosci. Abstr.* **20:**1471.

Sato, H., Fox, K., and Daw, N. W., 1989, Effect of electrical stimulation of locus coeruleus on the activity of neurons in the visual cortex, *J. Neurophysiol.* **62:**946–958.

Schoen, S. W., Leutenecker, B., Kreutzberg, G. W., and Singer, W., 1990, Ocular dominance plasticity and developmental changes of 5′-nucleotidase distributions in the kitten visual cortex, *J. Comp. Neurol.* **296:**379–392.

Shatz, C. J., and Stryker, M. P., 1988, Prenatal tetrodotoxin infusion blocks segregation of retinogeniculate afferents, *Science* **242:**87–89.

Sheu, F. S., Kasamatsu, T., and Routtenberg, A., 1990, Protein kinase C activity and substrate (F1/GAP-43) phosphorylation in developing cat visual cortex, *Brain Res.* **524:**144–148.

Stichel, C. C., and Singer, W., 1988, Localization of isoenzymes II/III of protein kinase C in the rat visual cortex (area 17), hippocampus and dentate gyrus, *Exp. Brain Res.* **72:**443–449.

Takahashi, M., Sugiyama, M., and Tsumoto, T., 1993, Contribution of NMDA receptors to tetanus-induced increase in postsynaptic Ca^{2+} in visual cortex of young rats, *Neurosci. Res.* **17:**229–239.

Wong, R. O. L., Meister, M., and Shatz, C. J., 1993, Transient period of correlated bursting activity during development of the mammalian retina, *Neuron* **11:**923–938.

Yuste, R., and Katz, L. C., 1991, Control of postsynaptic Ca^{++} influx in developing neocortex by excitatory and inhibitory neurotransmitters, *Neuron* **6:**333–344.

Deprivation Myopia and Emmetropization

I. Introduction

We pointed out in Chapter 6 that the eyeball grows in most people to be the correct size for the image to be in focus on the retina. This process is called emmetropization. Many infants are born hyperopic, and become emmetropic by 2–3 years of age. Some are born emmetropic and become myopic with age; that is, their eyeballs are too large for the power of the lens and the cornea, so that the image falls in front of the retina. A few are born myopic, and this is a condition that needs to be reversed early, because the eyeball can grow, but it cannot shrink.

The process of emmetropization requires a focused image on the retina. This point was underlined by a passing observation made by Hubel *et al.* (1975) in their work on monocular deprivation. In addition to the effects of monocular deprivation on the visual cortex, they discovered that the eyeball of the deprived eye was longer than normal (Fig. 13.1). The difference in length was over 1 mm, and the coating of the eyeball (sclera) on the posterior surface was thinned (Wiesel and Raviola, 1977). The effect was greater in young animals, and persisted for years after opening the eye again. When both eyes were closed, elongation of the eyeball was found in both eyes. Elongation of the eyeball depended on the diffusion of the image by the lid suture, rather than some mechanical effect of the lid suture on the eyeball, because the eyeballs were the same size when an animal with one eye closed was reared in the dark (Raviola and Wiesel, 1985). Thus, the focused image on the retina stops the eyeball from growing beyond the appropriate size. Disruption of emmetropization by diffusion of the image on the retina is called form-deprivation myopia.

A diffused image also causes myopia in humans. The largest study compared 12,000 normal patients to 73 patients with a variety of binocular visual abnormalities that prevented a clear image on the retina (Rabin *et al.*, 1981). The patients with binocular abnormalities were significantly more myopic (Fig. 13.2). Seven patients with monocular visual anomalies were also more myopic in the affected eye. Another study compared a pair of twins, one of whom had a congenital lens opacity (Johnson *et al.*, 1982). The eyeball was 2 mm longer in

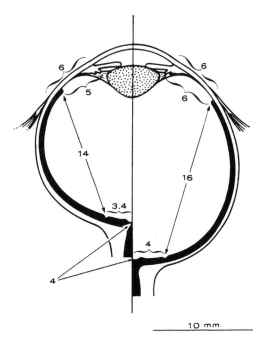

FIG. 13.1. Measurements illustrating the effects of neonatal lid fusion on various eye dimensions. Normal eye on the left, deprived eye on the right. Temporal halves of each retina are shown. Measurements in millimeters. Eyelids sutured from 2 weeks to 18 months of age. Reprinted with permission from Wiesel, T. N., and Raviola, E., 1977, Myopia and eye enlargement after neonatal lid fusion in monkeys, *Nature* **266**:66–68. Copyright 1977, MacMillan Magazines Limited.

the deprived eye of that twin, while the eyeballs of the normal twin differed by less than 0.2 mm. Although various theories have been proposed to account for these results, the present consensus is that the important factor in emmetropization is a clear image on the retina.

Control of emmetropization involves communication of signals from the retina to the growing wall of the eyeball. Form-deprivation myopia occurs in chicks after the optic nerve is cut (Troilo *et al.*, 1987; Wildsoet and Pettigrew, 1988), and in tree shrews when signals are prevented from reaching the central nervous system by blocking activity in retinal ganglion cells (Norton *et al.*,

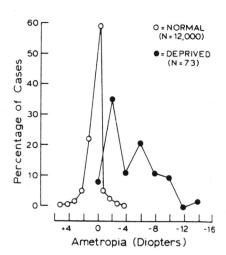

FIG. 13.2. Refractive error in normal and binocularly deprived eyes. The distribution of ametropia in binocularly deprived subjects is based on data from the more hyperopic of each subject's two eyes. Reprinted with permission from *Investigative Ophthalmology and Visual Science*, Rabin et al. (1981).

1994). The same result is obtained in one species of macaque, *Macaca mulatta* (Raviola and Wiesel, 1985). Thus, some signals affecting growth of the eyeball must emanate within the retina from bipolar or amacrine cells; signals from ganglion cells going to the central visual system are not necessary.

A dramatic illustration of local control is provided by experiments in chicks wearing translucent occluders placed so that the image is blurred on *part* of the retina (Wallman *et al.*, 1987). The sclera grows so that the part of the eyeball with a diffused image becomes myopic (the eyeball is elongated), while the part of the eyeball with a clear image remains emmetropic (Fig. 13.3). Refraction also varies from one part of the retina to another in normal animals. For example, in pigeons the upper part of the eyeball, which looks at the ground, is myopic in comparison with the lower part of the eyeball, which looks at more distant objects (Fitzke *et al.*, 1985). Local control of the size of the eyeball provides a mechanism to keep different parts of the retina in focus for objects at different distances, where the animal habitually looks at objects at different distances in different parts of the field of view.

Form-deprivation myopia implies a process of emmetropization; but does not prove it. For proof, one needs to show that the system becomes emmetropic after it is disturbed. Emmetropization as an active process is most easily studied in chicks, because their eyes show substantial growth over the first few weeks of life. Eyes covered with a negative lens grow more than usual, and eyes

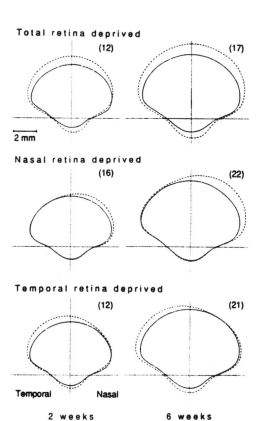

FIG. 13.3. Effect of form deprivation of part of the retina on the shape of the eye. When the nasal retina is deprived, this part of the eyeball grows, and when the temporal retina is deprived, that part of the eyeball grows. Solid lines show normal eyeballs, and interrupted lines deprived eyeballs. Results represent the average of a number of eyeballs, with the numbers given in parentheses. Reprinted with permission from Wallman *et al.*, *Science* **237**:73–77. Copyright 1987, American Association for the Advancement of Science.

covered with a positive lens grow less than usual (Schaeffel *et al.*, 1988; Irving *et al.*, 1992). When the lenses are taken off, the reverse occurs. Moreover, chicks that are reared with translucent occluders to produce form-deprivation myopia become emmetropic within a week or two after the occluders are removed (Troilo, 1990; see Fig. 13.4). In all cases, the growth of the eyeball tends to compensate for the treatment, so that the image becomes in focus on the retina.

Two changes in the shape of the eyeball have been shown to occur in the chick to produce emmetropization. One is an overall change in the length of the eyeball. The other is a change in the thickness of the layer of vascular tissue between the retina and the sclera, called the choroid. When the choroid thickens, it pushes the retina forward, which can compensate for the elongation of the eyeball that occurs in form-deprivation myopia (Fig. 13.5). In hyperopia, the choroid thins and the retina moves back, to compensate. Compensation for lack of focus in chicks involves a change in the thickness of the choroid, followed by a change in the length of the eyeball, during which the choroid tends to revert to its original thickness (Wallman *et al.*, 1995; see Fig. 13.6).

Given that a focused image can have a local effect on the growth of the eyeball, what might be the mechanism? One needs first a cell in the retina that can detect the difference between a focused image and an image that is diffused or out of focus. This cell then needs to release some substance, perhaps a neurotransmitter, and there needs to be a substantial change in the release for a focused image compared with an unfocused one. The substance or transmitter then needs to diffuse to the choroid or sclera without being taken up by cells along the way, or broken down by enzymes. Finally, there needs to be a mechanism whereby the substance or neurotransmitter affects the growth of the choroid and sclera.

Dopamine may be involved in form-deprivation myopia. Levels of dopamine and its metabolite DOPAC are reduced in the eyes of chicks with form-deprivation myopia (Stone *et al.*, 1989). Injection of the dopamine agonist

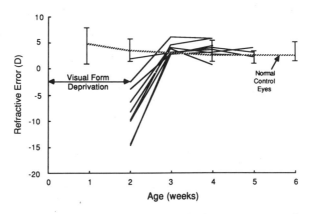

FIG. 13.4. Recovery from form-deprivation myopia in chicks. Myopia was induced by 2 weeks of visual form deprivation with translucent occluders. After the occluders were removed, the chicks became emmetropic within 1–3 weeks. Reprinted with permission from Troilo, D., 1990, Experimental studies of emmetropization in the chick, in: *Myopia and the Control of Eye Growth* (G. R. Bock and K. Widdows, eds.). John Wiley & Sons, Ltd., Chichester.

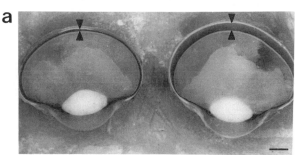

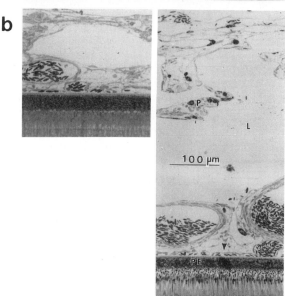

FIG. 13.5. Choroidal expansion in eyes recovering from myopia induced by form deprivation. (a) Unfixed hemisected eyes. Arrows indicate choroidal boundaries. (b) Sections of the posterior eye wall. Ch, choroid, delimited by arrows; L, lacuna; R, retina. Reprinted with kind permission from Wallman, J., Wildsoet, C., Xu, A., Gottlieb, M. D., Nickla, D., Marran, L., Krebs, W., and Christensen, A. M., 1995, Moving the retina: Choroidal modulation of refractive state, *Vision Res.* **35**:37–50. Copyright 1995, Elsevier Science, Ltd., The Boulevard, Langford Lane, Kidlington OX5 1GB, UK.

apomorphine reduces the extra growth of the eyeball during form deprivation. Moreover, there is a significant and dose-dependent effect on the axial length of the eyeball, but not on the equatorial diameter. Dopamine is released by amacrine cells in the retina, and can diffuse within it. Thus, cells containing dopamine could detect when images are out of focus, then dopamine could diffuse to the choroid and/or sclera to affect growth there. However, several more experiments will need to be done before this hypothesis is proved.

Another possible factor that has been studied is vasoactive intestinal peptide (VIP). VIP is found in a class of amacrine cells in the retina that comprise about 1% of the total. The level of VIP is increased during form deprivation that leads to myopia in monkeys (Stone *et al.*, 1988). Daily injections of VIP affect form-deprivation myopia in chicks, and some VIP antagonists eliminate it (Seltner and Stell, 1995). Moreover, VIP immunoreactivity is found in the choroid, where it could have an effect on choroidal blood flow.

The major biochemical changes associated with eye enlargement are an increase in DNA and protein synthesis and proteoglycan production in the cartilage of the sclera (Christensen and Wallman, 1991; Rada *et al.*, 1991). Regulation of proteoglycan production might be achieved by two growth factors

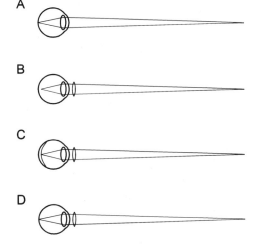

FIG. 13.6. Effect of thickness of choroid on refraction. (A) Image in focus on the retina in a young chick; (B) a positive lens places the image in front of the retina; (C) the choroid thickens to move the retina forward, and the image into focus again; (D) the optics of the eyeball change as it grows, and the choroid thins again to its original width.

that antagonize each other, such as basic fibroblast growth factor and transforming growth factor-beta, because these affect form-deprivation myopia appropriately for such a mechanism (Rohrer and Stell, 1994). However, we do not know if other growth factors have similar effects, where the various growth factors are located, what steps are involved in activation of the growth factors, and how the various growth factors affect proteoglycan production.

Thus, many experiments are still needed before we understand local control of eye growth. We need to know what the complete sequence of biochemical reactions is; which of the substances that have been investigated are part of this sequence of reactions, and which affect the reactions, but are not part of the sequence; whether the signal goes directly from the retina to the sclera, or the signal affects the choroid first, and the choroid in turn affects the sclera; and whether the sequence of reactions is the same in emmetropization and form-deprivation myopia.

Emmetropization involves the central nervous system, as well as local cues within the eyeball. All chicks can recover from form-deprivation myopia when their eyes are opened again, but the emmetropization is more accurate with an intact optic nerve than with the optic nerve sectioned (Troilo, 1990; Wildsoet and Wallman, 1995; see Fig. 13.7). Moreover, amblyopia, which is a cortical defect, may cause hyperopia. Some early evidence on this point came from Lepard (1975), who showed that the difference in refraction between normal and amblyopic eyes in strabismic amblyopes continues to increase for some time after the amblyopia develops (see Fig. 6.7). Monkeys with amblyopia produced by strabismus, or by blurred vision from a −10D lens in one eye, also become hyperopic, and the hyperopia develops after the amblyopia (Kiorpes and Wallman, 1995).

Emmetropization in primates is more complicated than in chicks. Because there is less room for the eyeball to grow, compensation may occur for a small amount of anisometropia, but not for a large amount (Hung *et al.*, 1994). Indeed, rearing with −10D lenses, for which a larger eyeball would compensate, actu-

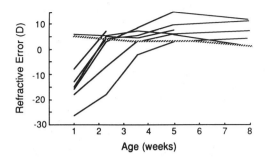

FIG. 13.7. Recovery from form-deprivation myopia overshoots the normal level in chicks with the optic nerve sectioned. Eyes were covered with translucent occluders for the first week. When occluders were taken off, recovery occurred over 1–3 weeks; however, all chicks had become hyperopic by the end of 5 weeks. Reprinted with permission from Troilo, D., 1990, Experimental studies of emmetropization in the chick, in: *Myopia and the Control of Eye Growth* (G. R. Bock and K. Widdows, eds.). John Wiley & Sons, Ltd., Chichester.

ally leads to a smaller one (Smith *et al.*, 1994). This may have occurred because contact lenses rather than spectacles were used. Alternatively, the primate visual system might interpret a large amount of hyperopia incorrectly. Interestingly, Nathan *et al.* (1985) found that refractive errors in children that affect primarily the fovea result in hyperopia, while refractive errors that affect primarily the periphery result in myopia. Perhaps the brain interprets the lack of well-focused images in the amblyopic eye as evidence of myopia, and therefore reduces elongation to compensate, producing hyperopia (see Kiorpes and Wallman, 1995).

The state of accommodation can also affect the whole process. There is a level of tonic accommodation which varies among individuals. A high level of tonic accommodation is found in corrected hyperopes, and a lack of tonic accommodation in late-onset myopes, as compared to emmetropes (McBrien and Millodot, 1987). It could be that the eyeball adjusts to the level of tonic accommodation found in different individuals. People with a high level of accommodation would tend to have the image focused in front of the retina, leading to compensation with a small eyeball, and people with a low level of accommodation would tend to have the image focused behind the retina, leading to a large eyeball.

II. Summary

Form-deprivation myopia differs from the other types of visual deprivation discussed in earlier chapters, in that it involves signals within the retina. Amblyopia from strabismus, anisometropia, and monocular deprivation, and meridional amblyopia from astigmatism, all involve changes that occur primarily in the visual cortex. Moreover, the mechanisms are different for amblyopia and form-deprivation myopia. So far, dopamine, peptides, and growth factors have been implicated in form-deprivation myopia, while glutamate receptors, calcium, second messengers, and synaptic proteins have been implicated in visual cortex changes.

At the functional level, there is a clear interaction between the two processes. Form deprivation leads to myopia, other optical changes can lead to hyperopia, and amblyopia can also lead to hyperopia over the long run. At the same time, hyperopia can lead to strabismus, which can lead to amblyopia. Moreover, myopia can lead to loss of contrast sensitivity. This emphasizes again the complexity of the visual system, and the interactions between its various components. The whole system is delicately balanced as it grows, and a deficit in any one of the components can lead to deficits in the others. We saw in earlier chapters how this is true in sensory and motor components of the system in the development of binocular vision. This chapter points out how it is also true in optical and sensory components of the system in development of correct focus on the retina.

References

Christensen, A. M., and Wallman, J., 1991, Evidence that increased scleral growth underlies visual deprivation myopia in chicks, *Invest. Ophthalmol. Vis. Sci.* **32:**2143–2150.

Fitzke, F. W., Hayes, B. P., Hodos, W., Holden, A. L., and Low, J. C., 1985, Refractive sectors in the visual field of the pigeon eye, *J. Physiol. (London)* **369:**33–44.

Hubel, D. H., Wiesel, T. N., and LeVay, S., 1975, Functional architecture of area 17 in normal and monocularly deprived macaque monkeys, *Cold Spring Harbor Symp. Quant. Biol.* **40:**581–589.

Hung, L. F., Smith, E. L., and Crawford, M. L. J., 1994, Infant monkey eyes can grow to compensate for an optically induced anisometropia, *Invest. Ophthalmol. Vis. Sci.* **35(Suppl.):**1805.

Irving, E. L., Sivak, J. G., and Callender, M. G., 1992, Refractive plasticity in the developing chick eye, *Ophthalmic Physiol. Opt.* **12:**448–456.

Johnson, C. A., Post, R. B., Chalupa, L. M., and Lee, T. J., 1982, Monocular deprivation in humans: A study of identical twins, *Invest. Ophthalmol. Vis. Sci.* **23:**135–138.

Kiorpes, L., and Wallman, J., 1995, Does experimentally-induced amblyopia cause hyperopia in monkeys? *Vision Res.* **35:**1289–1298.

Lepard, C. W., 1975, Comparative changes in the error of refraction between fixing and amblyopic eyes during growth and development, *Am. J. Ophthalmol.* **80:**485–490.

McBrien, N. A., and Millodot, M., 1987, The relationship between tonic accommodation and refractive error, *Invest. Ophthalmol. Vis. Sci.* **28:**997–1004.

Nathan, J., Kiely, P. M., Crewther, S. G., and Crewther, D. P., 1985, Disease-associated visual image degradation and spherical refractive errors in children, *Arch. Ophthalmol.* **62:**680–688.

Norton, T. T., Essinger, J. A., and McBrien, N. A., 1994, Lid-suture myopia in tree shrews with retinal ganglion cell blockade, *Vis. Neurosci.* **11:**143–154.

Rabin, J., Van Sluyters, R. C., and Malach, R., 1981, Emmetropization: A vision dependent phenomenon, *Invest. Ophthalmol. Vis. Sci.* **20:**561–564.

Rada, J. A., Thoft, R. A., and Hassell, J. R., 1991, Increased aggrecan (cartilage proteoglycan) production in the sclera of myopic chick, *Dev. Biol.* **147:**303–312.

Raviola, E., and Wiesel, T. N., 1985, An animal model of myopia, *N. Engl. J. Med.* **312:**1609–1615.

Rohrer, B., and Stell, W. K., 1994, Basic fibroblast growth factor (bFGF) and transforming growth factor beta (TGF-β) act as stop and go signals to modulate postnatal ocular growth in the chick, *Exp. Eye Res.* **58:**553–561.

Schaeffel, F., Glasser, A., and Howland, H. C., 1988, Accommodation, refractive error and eye growth in chickens, *Vision Res.* **28:**639–657.

Seltner, R. L. P., and Stell, W. K., 1995, The effect of vasoactive intestinal peptide on development of form deprivation myopia in the chick: A pharmacological and immunocytochemical study, *Vision Res.* **35:**1265–1270.

Smith, E. L., Hung, L. F., and Harwerth, R. S., 1994, Effects of optically induced blur on the refractive status of young monkeys, *Vision Res.* **34**:293–301.

Stone, R. A., Laties, A. M., Raviola, E., and Wiesel, T. N., 1988, Increase in retinal vasoactive intestinal peptide after eye lid fusion in primates, *Proc. Natl. Acad. Sci. USA* **85**:257–260.

Stone, R. A., Lin, T., Laties, A. M., and Iuvone, P. M., 1989, Retinal dopamine and form-deprivation myopia, *Proc. Natl. Acad. Sci. USA* **86**:704–706.

Troilo, D., 1990, Experimental studies of emmetropization in the chick, in: *Myopia and the Control of Eye Growth* (G. R. Bock and K. Widdows, eds.), Wiley, New York, pp. 89–102.

Troilo, D., Gottlieb, M. D., and Wallman, J., 1987, Visual deprivation causes myopia in chicks with optic nerve section, *Current Eye Res.* **6**:993–999.

Wallman, J., Gottlieb, M. D., Rajaram, V., and Fugate-Wentzek, L., 1987, Local retinal regions control local eye growth in chicks, *Science* **237**:73–77.

Wallman, J., Wildsoet, C., Xu, A., Gottlieb, M. D., Nickla, D., Marran, L., Krebs, W., and Christensen, A. M., 1995, Moving the retina: Choroidal modulation of refractive state, *Vision Res.* **35**:37–50.

Wiesel, T. N., and Raviola, E., 1977, Myopia and eye enlargement after neonatal lid fusion in monkeys, *Nature* **266**:66–68.

Wildsoet, C. F., and Pettigrew, J. D., 1988, Experimental myopia and anomalous eye growth patterns unaffected by optic nerve section in chickens: Evidence for local control of eye growth, *Br. J. Ophthalmol.* **3**:99–107.

Wildsoet, C., and Wallman, J., 1995, Choroidal and scleral mechanisms of compensation for spectacle lenses in chicks, *Vision Res.* **35**:1175–1194.

Conclusions

14

Future Studies

The third section of this book discusses what many people consider to be the current important question: What are the biochemical and molecular mechanisms of plasticity in the visual cortex? Although progress is being made in understanding mechanisms for LTP, progress regarding sensory-dependent plasticity in the visual cortex will inevitably be much slower, unless someone can show that the mechanisms are the same in the two cases, by some procedure that is less tedious than simply repeating everything done with LTP on sensory-dependent plasticity. In addition, there is some evidence of more than one type of LTP (dependent and not dependent on NMDA receptors), some evidence that LTP occurs where sensory-dependent plasticity does not, and some suggestions that there are anatomical changes in sensory-dependent plasticity that are not found with LTP.

Many of the results pertaining to this subject can be predicted: (1) that protein synthesis will be involved; (2) that the proteins produced will be those in membranes, in axonal and dendritic growth and retraction, and in synaptic processes, since complete processes and complete synapses are added and deleted; (3) that immediate early genes will be activated to control protein synthesis. Some useful information may be produced by quantitative measurements on these processes and their time course, but their existence seems fairly certain.

Much information will be generated by new techniques, such as subtractive hybridization to identify mRNAs whose levels are regulated during the critical period, and mice that have been treated so that a particular gene is absent (knock-out mice). Subtractive hybridization, like work on LTP, makes suggestions about what *might* be involved, rather than proves what *is* involved. The technique identifies mRNA that is expressed in substantially greater quantities in young animals than adults, and in dark-reared animals as compared with light-reared ones. Some of this mRNA will code for housekeeping proteins. Some of it may code for proteins directly involved in sensory-dependent plasticity. The greatest advantage of subtractive hybridization is that it can turn up suggestions that otherwise might not have been thought about.

Knock-out mice are mice that have been genetically engineered so that a particular gene is disrupted or completely deleted, such as a gene for one of the NMDA receptor subunits (Forrest *et al.*, 1994), or a gene for calcium–calmodulin-dependent kinase (CaM-KII) (Silva *et al.*, 1992). When a knock-out mouse is tested for the presence of sensory-dependent plasticity, a negative result is more significant than a positive result. For example, consider mice in which the gene for CaM-KII is absent. Ocular dominance plasticity is found in such mice (Gordon *et al.*, 1994). This suggests strongly that CaM-KII is not a critical component of the sequence of reactions involved in ocular dominance plasticity. On the other hand, if the experiment had turned out the other way (i.e., ocular dominance plasticity was not found in mice lacking CaM-KII), the result would have been difficult to interpret. Was ocular dominance plasticity abolished because CaM-KII is directly involved in ocular dominance plasticity, or because of an indirect effect? Knock-out mice seem likely to generate a long list, like Table 10-1, that will have to be evaluated by further experiments.

While experiments with these new molecular techniques are currently fashionable, there are a number of important questions remaining that need to be solved by anatomical and physiological techniques. In many cases, new anatomical and physiological techniques need to be devised before satisfactory answers can be given. During preparation of this book, the following questions struck me as being the most important. The first two questions will probably be of interest primarily to basic scientists. The other questions are mostly basic science questions that are important, in my opinion, for the treatment of amblyopia and strabismus. The list is a personal selection, and I am sure that others would come up with a different list.

I. What Are the Cellular Mechanisms for Changes in Orientation and Direction Deprivation?

The fundamental alterations involved in ocular dominance changes are believed to be the expansion and retraction of the terminals of excitatory neurons. At one time, it was thought that changes in inhibitory mechanisms might be involved (Duffy *et al.*, 1976). However, it turned out that inhibitory influences also contribute to the ocular dominance histogram in normal animals, to about the same extent as in monocularly deprived animals (Sillito *et al.*, 1981).

Unfortunately, how excitatory and inhibitory influences converge to create orientation and direction selectivity is controversial, with some people suggesting that inhibitory influences are the main contributor (Sillito, 1984; Eysel *et al.*, 1988), and others suggesting that excitatory influences alone can account for it (Ferster, 1987; Jagadeesh *et al.*, 1993). There is evidence that both excitatory and inhibitory influences contribute to direction selectivity in the rabbit retina (Wyatt and Daw, 1976; Ariel and Daw, 1982). According to my prejudice that, wherever there is a controversy in biology, both points of view eventually turn out to be correct, I would predict that both excitatory and inhibitory influences will be found to contribute to orientation and direction selectivity in the cat visual cortex. After all, orientation and direction selectivity are the main distinguishing features of visual cortex, and if GABA neurons do not contribute to orientation and direction selectivity, what are the GABA neurons there for? Once this controversy is settled with definitive evidence, we will be able to investigate which neurons are changing in sensory-dependent orientation and direction selectivity changes, and what the mechanisms are.

207

FUTURE STUDIES

II. What Governs the Segregation of Geniculocortical Afferents in Layer IV of the Visual Cortex?

The simple answer to this question is: electrical activity. However, it is a little more complicated than that. There is conjunction of electrical activity between neighboring cells within each eye, which should lead to dominance by one eye, and conjunction of activity between cells in one eye and corresponding cells in the other, which should lead to retention of binocular convergence. In the lateral geniculate nucleus, there is complete segregation of the left and right eye inputs into separate layers: conjunction of activity within each eye has been demonstrated, and complete lack of conjunction of activity between the eyes is assumed. Why does complete segregation not occur in layer IV of the visual cortex?

The process of segregation in the cortex starts when the synapses are first formed, between birth and 3 weeks of age. The simplest hypothesis is that there is some conjunction of activity within each eye, and little conjunction of activity between the eyes at 3 weeks of age, so that the cells start to become monocular. Then, between 3 and 6 weeks of age, conjunction of activity within each eye decreases, and conjunction of activity between the eyes increases, so that the cells do not become completely monocular. However, no one has ever done an experiment to see if this is what really happens. The experiment is feasible, and would be an interesting test of the Hebb postulate, as modified to take account of several presynaptic inputs.

III. The Cause of Congenital Esotropia

This subject was discussed at some length in Chapter 6, but a few more comments might be made here. In general, any factor that disturbs the feedback cycle between improvement of acuity, improvement of binocular fusion, and improvement in the accuracy of vergence movements can produce esotropia. As pointed out in Chapter 6, there are three theories about what might be happening in cases where the cause is unknown: failure of binocular fusion to overcome the tendency to prefer movement toward the nose; interruption of the cycle of improved fusion and vergence by the development of crossed stereopsis before uncrossed stereopsis; and misrouting of retinogeniculate projections at the optic chiasm.

The first theory is being actively studied, primarily by Tychsen (1993). At the present time, to my knowledge no one is doing experiments to test the second or third hypothesis. The second hypothesis would require a prospective study of a large number of children, of whom a small percentage would turn out to be esotropes, and measurement of the onset of stereoscopic acuity in each of them would be a time-consuming procedure. The third hypothesis is not currently a favored one, because many people believe that negative results using

VEPs have settled it. Nevertheless, the VEP is a crude technique, and more refined anatomical techniques might show a result where VEPs do not, if the material became available. Thus, the prime reason that the first hypothesis is being investigated, while the second and third are not, is that it is most likely that results will be obtained promptly from a study of the first hypothesis. In my opinion, the second and third hypotheses should be pursued as well.

IV. Development of Cellular Mechanisms for Stereoscopic Vision

Few investigators have studied physiological mechanisms of stereoscopic vision in the adult, and none in the developing animal. We know that there are "near" cells that respond to crossed disparity, and "far" cells that respond to uncrossed disparity (Poggio *et al.*, 1988). The exact location of these cells within the layers and columns of primary visual cortex in the primate has not been well determined, because of the difficulty of acquiring information on both physiology and anatomical location, which requires the use of a large number of animals; furthermore, considerable time must be spent training each animal to perform the task. A solid developmental study cannot be carried out until the organization in the adult is clear.

When the organization in the adult has been clarified, there are a number of questions that will need to be addressed in developing animals. When can cells sensitive to disparity first be found in physiological experiments? Do cells sensitive to crossed disparity appear before those sensitive to uncrossed disparity? At what level of processing are they found? Do they get input from left and right eyes that is precisely coordinated for orientation from the start, or is this initially sloppy, and then refined? Is the input from left and right eyes always the same as far as direction selectivity is concerned, or are there some cells that get input for leftward movement from one eye, and for rightward movement from the other? How does stereoscopic acuity develop?

After these questions are answered, one might be able to ask about the critical period for mechanisms of stereoscopic vision. More will be said about this below. It is clear that there are a long series of experiments that need to be done, because critical period questions cannot be addressed well until the developmental time course is determined, and the developmental time course cannot be so addressed until mechanisms of stereopsis in the adult are well worked out.

V. Mechanisms of Suppression in Strabismus

Very few papers have investigated the physiological mechanisms that may be involved in suppression of the image in one eye by the image in the other eye, which occurs in many cases of strabismus. In studying this question, one has to take account of the differences between esotropes and exotropes. For most esotropes, the eye that turns inward becomes amblyopic, and the image in this eye is also suppressed, unless the normal eye is open. For some exotropes, there is alternate fixation. The alternating exotrope looks at the image with the left eye, then with the right eye, then with the left eye, and so on. Generally speaking, alternation is associated with good acuity in both eyes, and constant suppression of one eye is associated with amblyopia in that eye. Constant suppression could involve a long-term or short-term mechanism, while suppression in alternators must involve a short-term mechanism.

Some authors have investigated the mechanism of suppression by electrical stimulation. Freeman and Tsumoto (1983) noticed that stimulation of the good eye was more likely to suppress stimulation of the deviating eye in esotropic cats than vice versa, and this was not noticed in exotropic cats. This point has not been noted by other authors. Moreover, none of the authors who have used electrical stimulation to investigate suppression have taken their investigations to the level of the single neuron, considered which neurons might be involved, or what the mechanisms might be. Is suppression a property of primary visual cortex, or higher areas as well? Is there an increased number of inhibitory GABA neurons driven by the good eye in esotropes? How can the system switch from suppression of one eye to the other eye in exotropes? What determines which eye is going to be the suppressor, and which the suppressed, and the rate of alteration? Are the mechanisms fundamentally the same, or fundamentally different between esotropes and alternating exotropes?

Sengpiel et al. (1994) have suggested that suppression in amblyopia may be an extension of the suppression that is found in normal people. Various forms of suppression occur normally. The term *masking* is used to refer to some of them. For example, if a letter is presented briefly, and shortly afterwards a surrounding circle is flashed on, the letter is not noticed. Contours interfere with the perception of neighboring contours. This is particularly true when one set of contours is in focus, and another set of contours is out of focus. Indeed, this is the reason why we do not notice afterimages in normal circumstances (Daw, 1962). Perhaps suppression in alternators is related to binocular rivalry, which occurs when two sharp representations reach the cortex, and constant suppression of one eye by the other is related to why we do not see afterimages, when a blurred representation is superimposed on a sharp one. However, this hypothesis leaves open the question of why esotropes develop one way, and some exotropes another.

Moreover, none of this discussion about whether suppression and masking in strabismus is like suppression and masking in normal people gets at the fundamental mechanisms involved, because the mechanisms of suppression in normal people are not understood at the cellular level. Does suppression involve the activation of GABA cells? Which GABA cells? How are they activated? At what level of the system does this occur? These are difficult investigations, but answers are needed.

VI. Where Is Anomalous Retinal Correspondence Located in the Primate?

We discussed in Chapter 7 how cells specific for anomalous retinal correspondence are found in the lateral suprasylvian cortex in the cat, which is secondary or tertiary visual cortex. The hypothesis is that anatomical rearrangements take place over a limited distance, and that the receptive fields in primary visual cortex are too small for compensation to occur there. Because the receptive fields are much larger in lateral suprasylvian cortex, a small distance in the cortex can compensate for a much larger distance on the retina.

In some cases, what seems to be anomalous retinal correspondence may be a rearrangement of the perception of the visual direction, rather than a rearrangement of the sensory pathways. Indeed, some ophthalmologists would claim that anomalous retinal correspondence in the strict sense does not exist. The experiments of Grant and Berman (1991) suggest that this is an extreme point of view, since Grant and Berman find cells specific for anomalous retinal correspondence at an early level of processing, even though it is not primary visual cortex. Nevertheless, several questions arise. Are there two definable entities—a rearrangement of sensory projections within the initial stages of sensory processing, as opposed to a change in the perception of direction—or more than two? In each case, what is the area within visual cortex, or perhaps visuomotor cortex, where the rearrangement takes place? What is the nature of the rearrangement, and the properties of the cells that get rearranged?

These questions need to be studied in primates for several reasons. First, the various regions of visual cortex are better defined in the primate than in the cat, even if the precise function of each region is a long way from being worked out. Second, primates can be trained to do both visual discrimination and visuomotor tasks, so that the physiology of the cortex can be investigated while they are doing a particular task. This behavioral training will be necessary to study the distinction between a rearrangement in sensory pathways and a rearrangement of perceived location. Third, the primate has a fovea, so its point of fixation is more precisely defined.

Unfortunately, there are a number of problems in designing such a study. One assumes that a rearrangement of connections in sensory pathways will only occur if the angle of deviation is fairly constant over a fairly long period of time, and not very large. This may be hard to arrange in a primate. More than one paradigm may have to be employed, to illustrate the large variety of situations that can occur in human strabismus. There will also be variability between animals. Consequently, a thorough study will be very long and time-consuming.

VII. The Development of a Precise Topographical Map

The time course of the development of a precise topographic map has not been studied, because the anatomical techniques are not available. Yet it is a most important question, when one considers the development of amblyopia. Just as ocular dominance changes are superimposed on the segregation of ocular dominance columns that takes place within layer IV of visual cortex, the development of amblyopia must be superimposed on the development of a precise topographic map. The general rule suggested in Chapter 9 is that there is a refinement of connections during development, and that the critical period for changing of connections lasts longer than the period over which the connections get refined during the normal course of development. In terms of this general rule, one would like to know when the geniculocortical connections initially become precise in normal animals.

As discussed in Chapter 5, the development of acuity depends largely on the development of the fovea, and of photoreceptors in the retina. Yet the development of a precise topographic map does affect acuity at certain periods during development. The comparison made by Jacobs and Blakemore (1988) shows that behavioral acuity is worse than acuity measured in the best cortical neurons until 2–3 months of age, and acuity measured in the best cortical neurons is worse than acuity in the best lateral geniculate neurons between 2 months and 1 year of age (see Fig. 5.2). Thus, one wants an anatomical technique that can be used to observe the precision of the projections between one level of the system and the next directly. Unfortunately, such a technique is not really available for measurements at the precision required. Hopefully one will be devised in the future.

One might add that we still do not know how the topography is organized in the first place. Is it related to molecular cues located in the subplate neurons? Is it related to some pattern in the timing of arrival of afferents to the cortex? These questions are still debated. However, the initial establishment of a coarse topographic map is not as important, as far as amblyopia is concerned, as the process of refinement of the map after it is initially formed.

VIII. Comparison of the Critical Periods for Amblyopia Binocularity, Anomalous Retinal Correspondence, and Stereoscopic Vision in Strabismus

We discussed in Chapter 9 how the critical period varies with the property being studied. The general rule suggested is that plasticity persists to a later time at higher levels of the system than at lower ones. The two best examples are that the critical period for ocular dominance changes ends later in output layers of primary visual cortex than in input layers, and that the critical period for orientation and direction, which is created in input layers of primary visual cortex, ends earlier than the critical period for ocular dominance changes, which is a property of output layers as well as input layers.

Establishment of the critical periods for the various deficits that can occur in strabismus is important for the treatment of those deficits. The current practice is based on a simple philosophy: the most important result is to have two eyes with good acuity, in case one of them is lost later in life, and to avoid diplopia. Thus, the eyes are aligned, acuity in the poor eye is improved with part-time patching, and binocular fusion is promoted with exercises. Little attention is paid to stereopsis, and there is only one case recorded in the entire history of ophthalmology of a strabismic child who was treated to reach binocular vision with adult stereoscopic acuity (Helveston, 1993).

Knowledge of the critical periods for amblyopia, for ocular dominance changes, for establishment of anomalous retinal correspondence, and for stereopsis, might reinforce this current practice. It could be that there is an inherent problem in the time course of these critical periods, such that one is never going to get perfect stereopsis in strabismic children, no matter how hard one tries. On the other hand, it could be that good stereopsis is possible, if one knows exactly when to intervene, and physician and parents are both very persistent. After all, most physicians used to consider treatment for congenital cataract to be an almost impossible task, while now it is known that the task is just very difficult, and good results can be achieved (see Chapter 8). The point is that basic scientists need to produce practical information to show whether a revised philosophy of treatment is justified.

Unfortunately, critical periods for these properties will be difficult to study. One needs to do the experiments in primates, because fine acuity and good stereopsis are not achieved in other mammals. As discussed above, development of stereopsis has not been studied, and the exact location of the cells subserving stereopsis is not known. It is hard to do a critical period study until these pieces of information are available. The same is true of anomalous retinal correspondence. There is more information on acuity, but even there some basic information on development is not available, for example, the time of establishment of a precise topographic map, as discussed above.

Design of experiments is complicated further by the wide variety of methods that can be used to create strabismus, and the difficulty of getting consistent results with any one of them. For example, one would like to produce a series of primates that have a constant comitant esotropia, say 10 diopters, for a fixed period of time, say 4 weeks, starting at a variety of different ages, say 4, 8, 12, 20, 40, and 80 weeks, and then study acuity, anomalous retinal correspondence, binocularity, and stereopsis at each age, and compare the results to those from normal animals of the same age. How does one do this? It is difficult to keep the esotropia constant and comitant, and to produce a sufficient number of animals so that all of the parameters can be studied. Nevertheless, the experiment is worthwhile, if we are to find out the best course of treatment for strabismus, and settle current controversies about the best age for intervention.

IX. Critical Periods at Higher Levels of the Visual System

We know that some visual perceptions are plastic forever. One of the most famous examples of this is that one can adjust to inversion of the whole world, as investigated by Stratton (1897) and Ivo Kohler (1964). In Stratton's experiments the world was inverted left–right and up–down with a telescope. In Kohler's experiments it was inverted either up–down, or left–right, with mirrors. In both cases, the subjects made substantial adaptations after a week or so. With up–down reversals, they learned to step up and down. With left–right reversals, they learned to ride a bicycle.

It was mostly visuomotor coordination and perception of movement that adapted. Some visual perceptions never did. This led to some strange results. For example, when presented with a picture of a vehicle moving from right to left, and asked what he saw, one subject replied that he saw a vehicle moving from right to left, but the letters on the license plate were reversed. More recently, Held (1965) has shown that visuomotor coordination can adapt over a period of minutes. This is probably adaptation of the motor system, perhaps in the cerebellum, rather than an adaptation in the visual system (Harris, 1965).

These psychological experiments provide most intriguing food for thought for critical periods at higher levels of the visual system. However, it will be difficult to study them before the functions of the 30 or so areas in cortex dealing with vision have been defined. Most likely there are adaptations more complicated than closing off one eye, and less global than turning the whole world upside down, that affect areas somewhere between primary visual cortex and the cerebellum. Such adaptations in monkeys might be expected to have a critical period ending somewhere after 1 year, when the critical period for ocular dominance changes ends, and death, when the critical period for visuomotor adaptations ends.

X. Conclusion

My final conclusion is that we have learned an enormous amount about plasticity in the visual system over the last 30 years. Study of the clinical features of the problem in humans goes back into ancient history, but the concept that early intervention is important did not become apparent until the middle of the 20th century. Study of the anatomical and physiological features goes back to the work of Wiesel and Hubel in the mid-1960s. The fundamental properties are now understood, largely as a result of their work, but many details that are important for clinical treatment remain to be worked out. Study of the mechanisms is currently a very active area of research, and owes a lot to results obtained from experiments on long-term potentiation. I have enjoyed being a part of this exciting field of research over the last 30 years, and expect that the next 30 years will be equally exciting, with work that will lead to improvements in clinical treatment, as well as a deep understanding of the mechanisms that guide visual development.

References

Ariel, M., and Daw, N. W., 1982, Pharmacological analysis of directionally sensitive rabbit retinal ganglion cells, *J. Physiol. (London)* **324:**161–185.

Daw, N. W., 1962, Why after-images are not seen in normal circumstances, *Nature* **196:**1143–1145.

Duffy, F. H., Snodgrass, S. R., Burchfield, J. L., and Conway, J. L., 1976, Bicuculline reversal of deprivation amblyopia in the cat, *Nature* **260:**256–257.

Eysel, U. T., Muche, T., and Worgotter, F., 1988, Lateral interactions at direction-selective striate neurones in the cat demonstrated by local cortical inactivation, *J. Physiol. (London)* **399:**657–675.

Ferster, D., 1987, Origin of orientation-selective EPSPs in simple cells of cat visual cortex, *J. Neurosci.* **7:**1780–1791.

Forrest, D., Yuzaki, M., Soares, H. D., Ng, L., Luk, D. C., Sheng, M., Stewart, C. L., Morgan, J. I., Connor, J. A., and Curran, T., 1994, Targeted disruption of NMDA receptor 1 gene abolishes NMDA response and results in neonatal death, *Neuron* **13:**325–338.

Freeman, R. D., and Tsumoto, T., 1983, An electrophysiological comparison of convergent and divergent strabismus in the cat: Electrical and visual activation of single cortical cells, *J. Neurophysiol.* **49:**238–253.

Gordon, J. A., Silva, A., Morris, R., Stewart, C., Silver, I., Tokugawa, Y., and Stryker, M. P., 1994,

Plasticity in mouse visual cortex: Critical period and effects of αCaMKII and Thy-I mutations, *Soc. Neurosci. Abstr.* **20**:465.

Grant, S., and Berman, N. E. J., 1991, Mechanism of anomalous retinal correspondence: Maintenance of binocularity with alteration of receptive-field position in the lateral suprasylvian (LS) visual area of strabismic cats, *Vis. Neurosci.* **7**:259–281.

Harris, C. S., 1965, Perceptual adaptation to inverted, reversed, and displaced vision, *Psychol. Rev.* **72**:419–444.

Held, R., 1965, Plasticity in sensory-motor systems, *Sci. Am.* **213**:84–94.

Helveston, E. M., 1993, The origins of congenital esotropia, *J. Pediatr. Ophthalmol. Strabismus* **30**:215–232.

Jacobs, D. S., and Blakemore, C., 1988, Factors limiting the postnatal development of visual acuity in the monkey, *Vision Res.* **28**:947–958.

Jagadeesh, B., Wheat, H. S., and Ferster, D., 1993, Linearity of summation of synaptic potentials underlying direction selectivity in simple cells of the cat visual cortex, *Science* **262**:1901–1904.

Kohler, I., 1964, The formation and transformation of the perceptual world. (tr. H. Fiss), *Psychol. Issues* **3(4)**.

Poggio, G. F., Gonzalez, F., and Krause, F., 1988, Stereoscopic mechanisms in monkey visual cortex: Binocular correlation and disparity selectivity, *J. Neurosci.* **8**:4531–4550.

Sengpiel, F., Blakemore, C., Kind, P. C., and Harrad, R., 1994, Interocular suppression in the visual cortex of strabismic cats, *J. Neurosci.* **14**:6855–6871.

Sillito, A. M., 1984, Functional considerations of the operation of GABAergic inhibitory processes in the visual cortex, in: *Cerebral Cortex* (E. G. Jones and A. Peters, eds.), Plenum Press, New York, pp. 91–117.

Sillito, A. M., Kemp, J. A., and Blakemore, C. 1981, The role of GABAergic inhibition in the cortical effects of monocular deprivation, *Nature* **291**:318–320.

Silva, A. J., Stevens, C. F., Tonegawa, S., and Wang, Y., 1992, Deficient hippocampal long-term potentiation in α-calcium-calmodulin kinase II mutant mice, *Science* **257**:201–206.

Stratton, G. M., 1897, Vision without inversion of the retinal image, *Psychol. Rev.* **4**:241–360.

Tychsen, L., 1993, Motion sensitivity and the origins of infantile strabismus, in: *Early Visual Development, Normal and Abnormal* (K. Simons, ed.), Oxford University Press, London, pp. 364–390.

Wyatt, H. J., and Daw, N. W., 1976, Specific effects of neurotransmitter antagonists on ganglion cells in rabbit retina, *Science* **191**:204–205.

Glossary

AC/A ratio   This ratio represents the amount of convergence that occurs for a specific amount of accommodation. In normal people, if one refocuses from an object 10 feet away to an object 3 feet away, the amount of convergence is appropriate so that the object at 3 feet will fall on corresponding parts of the retinas. This is a normal AC/A ratio. Some people may converge too much (a high AC/A ratio) and others may converge too little (a low AC/A ratio). See *near response.*

Accommodation   Change in the shape of the lens to focus images at different distances on the retina. Contraction of the circular ciliary muscle around the margin of the lens makes the lens more convex to focus nearby objects. Relaxation of the ciliary muscle, and tension in the zonule fibers that support the lens makes the lens flatter, to focus objects far away.

Acuity   The ability to detect fine detail. It is tested in a physician's office by asking the subject to read a line of letters (Snellen acuity). Someone who can only read a line at 20 feet (6 meters) that a person with normal adult acuity can read at 60 feet (18 meters) is said to have an acuity of 20/60 or 6/18, which is one third of normal. People with acuity of less than 20/200 (10% of normal) after correction of their optics are legally blind.

   Acuity can also be tested with a grating of black and white lines of equal width. The subject is asked to detect the orientation of the lines in the grating, compared with a uniform gray area of the same shape and overall luminance. The limit of acuity is the finest grating that can be detected. The result is expressed in cycles per degree, where one cycle is the width of one black plus one white line, and one calculates how many cycles can be detected in 1° of arc from the point of view of the observer. Most people can see 30 cycles/degree, and this is equivalent to a Snellen acuity of 20/20.

   Another test that can be used with some people who cannot read is the Landolt C. C's are arranged in one of four orientations. The subject is asked to detect whether the gap in the C is on the left, right, top, or bottom, and the size of the letters is reduced until the subject can no longer detect the position of the gap.

Adaptation   This word has been used to describe a large variety of phenome-

215

na. In general, it means that the state of the visual system changes to become more or less sensitive to some class of stimuli.

Light adaptation is the process of becoming used to a higher level of illumination, so that one is most sensitive to objects near this level of illumination. While the visual system is able to respond over 12 log units of brightness, at any one time the system only responds to 2 log units. For objects that are not colored, the brightest object is white, an object 2 log units less bright than this is black, and in between are shades of gray. Light adaptation occurs rapidly, in seconds, or less for moderate changes of illumination.

Dark adaptation is the process of becoming more sensitive to dim objects. It is determined by the percentage of molecules of the rod photopigment, rhodopsin, that are bleached. Bleached molecules send signals up the visual pathway that are equivalent to a background of light, so that an object that is much dimmer than this background cannot be seen. Rhodopsin regenerates with a slow time course—the time constant is about 15 min—so that one cannot see clearly in very dim light until 30–45 minutes has passed.

Light and dark adaptation depend on processes that occur in the retina. Cells at higher levels of the system can adapt to more complicated stimuli (see *aftereffects*).

Afferents Axons that come into the nucleus or area being described.

Aftereffects Aftereffects occur because of adaptation of cells at higher levels of the visual system. The best known are probably the direction-selective aftereffects. In the waterfall phenomenon, after staring at a waterfall, the bank nearby will appear to move upward. In the spiral aftereffect, after staring at the center of a rotating spiral, when the rotation stops, it will appear as though the spiral is rotating in the opposite direction. These aftereffects are caused by adaptation of direction-selective cells in the visual cortex.

Another example is the tilt aftereffect. In the tilt aftereffect, the subject stares at a set of lines tilted to the left for a few minutes, then transfers his/her attention to a set of vertical lines. The vertical lines appear to be tilted to the right for a short time.

Anisometropia A difference in focus for the two eyes, so that when one eye accommodates for an object to be in focus on the retina of that eye, the object is out of focus for the retina of the other eye. Anisometropia is a problem because accommodation is consensual; that is, the two eyes accommodate together, and cannot accommodate separately in normal people.

Anomalous retinal correspondence If the connections between one of the retinas and some part of cortex are rewired during development, so that the fovea of one eye, and some point that is not the fovea in the other eye, project to the same place in the cortex, then the subject has anomalous retinal correspondence. This occurs in strabismus, but only rarely, because it requires that the angle of strabismus be constant (comitant) over a substantial period of time, so that the new connections can be established.

Aphakia This is the absence of a lens in the eye. It occurs in cataract, when the lens is taken out. There are three resulting optical problems. First, the eye needs an additional lens to focus (a contact lens or spectacles), but this leads to images that are different sizes on the retina if the additional lens is outside the eyeball. Second, another lens is required to avoid the difference in magnification, unless an intraocular lens implant is used. Third, the eye cannot accommodate.

Astigmatism   A cylindrical component in the optics of the eye, so that when lines in one orientation are in focus, lines along the orthogonal orientation are out of focus.

Binocular fusion   For images that fall on corresponding points of the two retinas, the images will be fused into a single perception in the visual cortex. There can be a small mismatch, and the images will still be fused. For example, an object that is farther away than the plane of fixation will fall on noncorresponding points of the two retinas, but it will be seen as single and distant. See *Panum's fusional area*.

Blob   This is the term for areas in layers III and II of primate striate cortex that stain heavily for cytochrome oxidase, which is a marker for increased metabolic activity. The blobs are in the center of ocular dominance columns, and contain a high percentage of color-coded cells.

Cataract   A lens that is opaque or cloudy. Cataracts are most frequently found in old people, but they can also be congenital. There are a variety of causes, such as rubella (German measles). If the cloudiness is confined to the center of the lens, then a clear image can be obtained through the edge of the lens. When the cataract covers the whole lens, then the image on the retina is diffused.

Choroid   A layer of vascular tissue between the sclera and pigment epithelium.

Comitant strabismus   A form of strabismus where the eyes move together, so that there is a fairly constant angle between the direction of view of the two eyes. Congenital esotropia is usually comitant.

Contrast sensitivity   Sensitivity to contrast is a measure of the minimum contrast that can be seen. Generally speaking, an object can be detected if it differs from the background by more than 1%. However, this depends on the size of the object and the overall illumination. Contrast sensitivity is generally measured with gratings where both spatial frequency and contrast can be varied. It is usually expressed as

$$\frac{L_{max} + L_{min}}{L_{max} - L_{min}}$$

where L_{max} is the luminance of the lighter stripes and L_{min} is the luminance of the darker stripes. Thus, the contrast sensitivity for a 1% difference in luminance is ~ 200.

Cortical plate   As the cerebral cortex develops, young cells migrate out from the ventricular zone through the subventricular and intermediate zones to form the cortical plate. The cortical plate consists of cells that have reached their final destination, and cells migrating through, until all layers of the cortex are formed.

Diplopia   Double vision. The condition is usually binocular, occurring with strabismus when the image in the crooked eye is not suppressed. In rare cases of anomalous retinal correspondence, it can be monocular. In these cases, the new fixation point in the crooked eye is connected to central vision in the cortex, the original connections still exist, and the signals traveling down the original connections are not suppressed.

Disparity   Disparity occurs when an image falls on noncorresponding parts of the two retinas. It happens whenever there is an object at a different distance from the object being fixated. For objects nearer than the fixation point, the lines of sight from the two eyes cross each other between the eyes and the plane of fixation: this is called *crossed disparity*. For an object farther than the fixation point, the lines of sight from the two eyes do not cross each other, and this is called *uncrossed disparity*.

Eccentricity   The field of view comprises the fixation point, and an area out to approximately 90° away from the fixation point. Eccentricity is a measure of distance away from the fixation point in the field of view, usually expressed in degrees of angle. It can also be the distance from the fovea in the retina.

Efferents   Axons that leave the nucleus or area being considered.

Electroretinogram (ERG)   This is a measure of the sum of all the electrical activity in the retina measured from electrodes outside the retina. In humans, it can be measured between an electrode placed on the sclera and an electrode placed on the skin. There are several components of the ERG: the **a** wave, coming from photoreceptors; the **b** wave, coming from cells in the inner nuclear layer, and summed by the Muller cells, which are the glial cells of the retina; and the **c** wave, coming from the pigment epithelium.

Emmetropia   The visual state where images are in focus on the retina.

Esotropia   Strabismus where one eye turns inward. It can be congenital, probably from a variety of causes that remain to be pinned down. It can occur in young children from hyperopia, and in older children from a variety of causes.

Exotropia   Strabismus where one eye turns outward.

Fixation   The process of looking directly at an object. In normal people, this means that the image of the object falls on the foveas of the two eyes. Since images that are stationary on the retina disappear (because signals in the visual cortex are transient), the process of fixation actually involves slow eye movements away from the object, with small fast movements (microsaccades) that tend to bring the image back to the fovea.

FPL   Forced-choice preferential looking technique. An infant faces two displays. An observer looks at the infant from behind a screen, and is forced to record whether the infant is looking at the left display or the right display. If the records from the observer show that the infant looks at one display more than the other on more than 75% of the observations, the infant is said to be able to discriminate between the displays. Some criterion level other than 75% may be chosen.

Fusion   See *binocular fusion*.

Grating acuity   See *acuity*.

Habituation   When a stimulus is presented repeatedly, the response may decrease. If it does, this is called habituation. Habituation is particularly noticeable in the response from cells in the visual cortex in young animals. Sometimes one may have to wait several seconds between stimuli, if each response to the stimulus is to be as large as the first.

Hypercolumn   The cortex is organized in a columnar fashion; that is, cells on a line perpendicular to the surface of the cortex tend to have similar properties. There are columns in primary visual cortex in primates for ocular dominance, orientation, and color, organized around the blobs, which are primarily for color. Thus, there is a small module, approximately 1 × 1 mm, which analyzes a small area of the field of view for all of these parameters. This module is called a hypercolumn. Next door will be another hypercolumn, analyzing a neighboring part of the field of view. The size of a hypercolumn tends to be constant as one moves across the cortex. However, the area of field of view that it analyzes increases with eccentricity (the distance from the fovea). Near the fovea, a hypercolumn analyzes approximately 0.3° of the field of view, and 20° away from the fovea, a hypercolumn analyzes 1.5° of the field of view. Thus, the part of the visual field that falls on the fovea is analyzed in greater detail than the rest of the visual field.

Hyperopia   Where the image is consistently behind the retina, because the eyeball is too small for the focusing power of the cornea and lens, and there is not enough accommodative power in the system to overcome this. It can be corrected with convex lenses.

Hypertropia   Strabismus where the deviating eye looks upward.

Hypotropia   Strabismus where the deviating eye looks downward.

Incomitant strabismus   Strabismus where one eye moves and the other moves much less, or not at all. An obvious example occurs when the muscle that moves the eye outward is paralyzed.

Increment threshold   Measurement of the smallest increment in luminance that can be seen against a background. This depends on the size of the object, just as contrast sensitivity depends on spatial frequency.

LTP   Long-term potentiation. This is a long-term change in the efficacy of transmission across a synapse, as a result of high-frequency stimulation of the input to the synapse. LTP is believed to underlie some forms of memory, primarily because it is a prominent phenomenon in the hippocampus, and people with lesions of the hippocampus have deficits in short-term memory.

Masking   The visibility of an object can be decreased by an object placed beside it (spatial masking), or by another object seen after it (temporal masking). For example, if a letter is flashed on the screen, followed a moment later by a circle around it, the letter may not be seen. Similarly, letters in a line are less visible than a letter by itself (the crowding phenomenon). Both temporal and spatial masking occur in normal people.

Meridional amblyopia   The form of amblyopia that occurs with astigmatism. Lines oriented along the axis of good vision are less visible than lines oriented along the orthogonal axis, if the astigmatism is maintained, and not corrected, for several years before the age of 7.

Microsaccade   A small saccadic eye movement made to keep the image near the fovea during the process of fixation.

Myopia   Where the eyeball is too long for the power of the cornea and the lens, so that the image is consistently focused in front of the retina.

Near response   Term used to refer to the three changes that occur when the eyes refocus on a near object: the lens accommodates, the eyes converge, and the pupil contracts.

Nystagmus   A jerky or undulating movement of the eyes. In normal people, nystagmus can be stimulated by an environment moving around the person (optokinetic nystagmus, or OKN) or by activation of the vestibular system (vestibular nystagmus). In these two cases, there is a slow movement of the eyes, designed to keep the image stationary on the retina, followed by a saccade-like fast movement to bring the eyes back to a central position. Nystagmus can also be pathological, in patients who have amblyopia and lose good fixation. In this case, the nystagmus is usually a slow wandering of the eyes from side to side (pendular nystagmus), rather than an alternation of slow and fast movements.

Object color constancy   Objects tend to appear the same color under different sources of illumination. For example, a blue sweater will appear blue in both tungsten light and daylight, and a yellow sweater will appear yellow in both of those sources of illumination, even though tungsten light is yellowish and daylight is bluish.

OKN   See *nystagmus*.

Orthotropia   The two eyes look in the same direction, and the image of the object being fixated falls on the foveas of the two retinas.

Panum's fusional area   Images falling on noncorresponding parts of the two retinas can be fused, presumably by the cells in the visual cortex that are sensitive to disparity. However, there is a limit to this. The area in one eye that can be fused with a point in the other is known as Panum's fusional area. It is approximately 15 minutes wide near the fovea, and gets larger with eccentricity. Images falling outside Panum's area will produce diplopia if not suppressed.

Parallel processing   Term referring to the fact that different aspects of visual perception are processed in parallel with each other. For example, there are cells that respond to objects brighter than the background and cells that respond to objects darker than the background, among bipolar and ganglion cells in the retina, cells in the lateral geniculate nucleus, and simple cells in the visual cortex. The two types of signal are separated from each other after processing by the photoreceptors, and do not come together again until the visual cortex is reached. Thus, there is little intermingling between the two cell types along the way.

Prospective study   A study where a population is investigated for factors that may affect a disease or condition, starting before the onset of the disease or condition.

Pursuit eye movements   Also known as *smooth pursuit eye movements*. These occur when the eyes are following an object. The eyes cannot move smoothly, unless there is an object to be followed. If a person is asked to move his or her eyes smoothly from one point to another, what actually happens is a series of saccades. Smooth pursuit eye movements are essentially fixation on a moving object.

Quantum catch   The number of quanta of light caught by a photoreceptor, compared with the number of quanta falling on the photoreceptor. The quantum catch depends on the length of the photoreceptor, whether the light comes in parallel to the photoreceptor or at an angle, the density of pigment, how much of the pigment is bleached, and how the inner segment of the photoreceptor funnels light into the outer segment.

Reflection spectrum   One can measure the percentage of light reflected by an object for each wavelength in the visible spectrum. This is the reflection spectrum of the object. Red objects reflect a lot of red wavelengths (620–700 nm), green objects reflect a lot of green wavelengths (520–560 nm), and blue objects reflect a lot of blue wavelengths (420–480 nm). The light that reaches the eye from an object is the product of the wavelengths emitted by the source of illumination, and the reflection spectrum of the object. Generally speaking, the color of an object in a multicolored scene is predicted better by its reflection spectrum than by the composition of wavelengths that reach the eye from it. Thus, object color constancy occurs.

Refraction   The process of measuring the optics of the eye for correction with spectacles or contact lenses.

Resolution limit   The limit of the finest detail that can be seen, i.e., the limit of acuity.

Retrospective study   A study where a population is investigated for factors that may affect a disease or condition, starting after the onset of the disease or condition. Bias is much more likely in a retrospective study than in a prospective study, and data for the time before the disease or condition started may not be reliable.

Reverse suture   Procedure where the eyelids of one eye are sutured closed for a period of time, then opened, and the eyelids of the other eye are sutured closed.

Rivalry   Where different images fall on the two retinas, and the percept alternates between the two. For example, there may be horizontal lines falling on the left retina, and vertical lines falling on the right retina, and the perception will alternate between horizontal lines and vertical lines.

Saccade   A fast eye movement designed to move the line of sight to a new and interesting object in the periphery of the field of view. Saccadic eye movements are ballistic, i.e., once one is started it cannot be interrupted, and a period of 200 msec is necessary before another one can be started. Large saccadic eye movements are very fast—up to 800° per second.

Saturation discrimination Discrimination of a color from a more or less saturated color of the same hue, i.e., how much white needs to be added or subtracted before one can notice the difference.

Sclera The outside coat of the eyeball.

Scotoma A blind spot caused by a lesion in the visual pathways. A lesion of the retina or optic nerve will affect one eye only, so the scotoma will be monocular. A lesion of the optic tract, lateral geniculate nucleus, optic radiations, or visual cortex will affect both eyes, so the scotoma will be binocular (see Fig. 2.3).

Sign-conserving synapse, and sign-reversing synapse With a sign-conserving synapse, the response in presynaptic and postsynaptic cells has the same sign. If the presynaptic cell is hyperpolarized, then the postsynaptic cell will also be hyperpolarized. If the presynaptic cell is depolarized, so will the postsynaptic cell. At a sign-reversing synapse, hyperpolarization of the presynaptic cell leads to depolarization of the postsynaptic cell, and depolarization of the presynaptic cell leads to hyperpolarization of the postsynaptic cell. The transmitter at sign-conserving synapses is excitatory, and the transmitter at sign-reversing synapses is inhibitory. For hyperpolarization in the presynaptic cell to act on the postsynaptic cell, there has to be spontaneous activity and continuous release of transmitter at the synapse.

All of this is pretty obvious, but the terminology has arisen because photoreceptors hyperpolarize in response to light. Thus, depolarizing bipolar cells are excited by light, but inhibited by the transmitter released from photoreceptors, because the hyperpolarization in the photoreceptors depolarizes the bipolar cell across the sign-reversing synapse between them. It is easier to say that depolarizing bipolar cells are excited by light through a sign-reversing synapse, than to say that they are excited by light through an inhibitory synapse.

Simultaneous color contrast The tendency for an object surrounded by a different color to take on a color opposite to the surroundings. Thus, a gray spot in a red surround tends to look greenish, in a green surround reddish, in a blue surround yellowish, and in a yellow surround bluish.

Snellen acuity See *acuity*.

Spatial frequency The periodicity of a periodic object such as a grating. Expressed in terms of cycles per degree (see *contrast sensitivity*).

Spatial uncertainty Uncertainty about the location of an object. This can be tested by asking a subject to line up an object between two other objects above and below it (see Fig. 8.3); by asking a subject to place objects equidistant on various sides of a marker in the center (see Fig. 8.13); and by vernier stimuli (see Fig. 3.7).

Spectral sensitivity Sensitivity to various different wavelengths compared with each other. In the dark-adapted state, the spectral sensitivity curve follows the sensitivity of the rod pigment, rhodopsin. In the light-adapted state, it follows the envelope of the curves for the red- and green-absorbing cone pigments, with a smaller contribution from the blue-absorbing cone pigment.

Stereopsis Stereoscopic depth perception depends on disparity. The cells in the visual cortex sensitive to crossed disparity detect near objects, and lead to a perception of nearness and possibly convergent eye movements. The cells sensitive to uncrossed disparity detect far objects. Stereoscopic acuity, like vernier acuity, is much better than grating acuity. Observers with very good stereoscopic vision can discriminate two objects that are 0.02 inch apart in depth at a distance of 6 feet. This corresponds to 2 seconds of arc from the point of view of the observer.

Strabismus   Condition where the two eyes look in different directions. Colloquially known as cross-eyed, or squint.

Subplate cells   Cells found below the cortical plate during development. They are generated before cells that are destined to end up in layers II–VI of the cortex. Most of them die soon after birth. The remnants are called interstitial cells.

Successive color contrast   After staring at an object for a period of time, the succeeding object to be observed will be tinged with the complementary color. For example, looking at gray after staring at red will make the gray appear greenish.

Suppression   Term used to refer to suppression of the image in one eye by the image in the other eye. It is the visual system's mechanism to avoid diplopia. Suppression can be alternating, as in binocular rivalry or alternate fixation by an exotrope, or it can be continual suppression of one eye by the other, as in suppression of the image in the amblyopic eye by the straight eye in congenital esotropes.

Temporal frequency   This term is usually applied to a grating where the stripes are flickered between black and white, i.e., the white stripes become black and the black stripes become white several times a second. The rate of flicker can be increased until the flicker is no longer noticed. The frequency at which this happens depends on the contrast of the stimulus. Consequently, one can construct a temporal sensitivity curve, just as one constructs a contrast sensitivity curve for spatial frequency.

Tilt aftereffect   See *aftereffects.*

VEP   Visually evoked potential. This is measured from electrodes placed on the scalp over the visual cortex. To get much of a potential, one needs a stimulus that will activate many cells in the visual cortex in synchrony with each other. One stimulus commonly used is a checkerboard, with the squares on the checkerboard flickering between black and white.

Vergence   Eye movements by which the eyes look at objects at different distances—convergence for nearby objects, and divergence for distant objects. These are slow eye movements. They are conjugate, in the sense that the eyes move together (all eye movements—saccades, smooth pursuit eye movements, and vergence movements—are conjugate).

Vernier acuity   This is the ability to detect a break in a line. It can be measured with a grating, as shown in Fig. 3.7, or a single line that is essentially one line in that figure. Vernier acuity is approximately 10% of grating acuity: while grating acuity is 2 minutes of arc in normal people, vernier acuity is 12 seconds of arc.

Index

Entries in the Glossary are referred to with the letter g.